A fortune in vials: A pharmacist's pursuit

By Samar Jamil

Introduction:

Alex and mark are friends since they were at the university , they grown In poor families and they were suffering until they finish their bachelor of pharmacy , they were working to support their families while studying , now Alex is 28 years old and mark is 30 years old , they believe in hope , they have the inspiration and ambitious to get what they dreamed about, after several years they decided to go to Canada to get more opportunities and get a better life, they know it's a huge change and its going to be so hard for them to do that alone , the only thing who helped them is Simon , they get referred to Simon by other friend to help them , their degree is like a weapon for them with fluent English .

our friends set a goal to change their life and want to be rich in 10 years.

is it going to be easy?

What kind of obstacles will stand in their way?

Are they able to do it?

Let's find out …...

The beginning

Alex wiped the sweat from his brow as he and Mark trudged along the bustling streets of Toronto, the city's summer heat reflecting off the concrete like waves of invisible fire. The weight of their pharmacy degrees felt heavier with each passing day in this new country, barely two months since their arrival, when Alex turned to Mark, determination etching his features.

"Ten years," Alex said resolutely. "We'll make our fortune here in ten years. But first things first—we need jobs."

The bell above the door jangled as Alex and Mark pushed their way into the warm interior of Tim Hortons. The smell of coffee and baked goods wrapped around them like a comforting blanket, but they barely noticed. They had one thing on their minds: securing any job that could put them one step closer to their dreams of wealth.

"Man, I'll even take a gig flipping burgers at this point," Mark muttered, scanning the crowded space for an empty table.

"Same," Alex agreed, his gaze falling on Simon, who was busy wiping down the counter with a practiced hand. He recognized the man from a few encounters in the past—always behind this counter, always with a ready smile.

"Hey, Simon!" Alex called out, waving to catch the man's attention. Mark followed suit with a nod of acknowledgment.

Simon looked up, his face breaking into a friendly grin. "Alex, Mark! What brings you guys here?"

"Job hunt," Mark said, sliding onto a stool at the counter. "You know anyone hiring?"

"Actually," Simon began, tossing the rag over his shoulder, "we might need some extra hands around here. tell me about you, guys."

"Yes," Alex replied, relief buoying his spirits.

Mark nodded, his own resolve mirroring Alex's. Fluent in English, they had anticipated fewer barriers, yet the job market proved stubborn. Day after scorching day, they combed through listings, pounded the pavement, and shook countless hands until, their persistence met opportunity.

"Simon," the man had introduced himself outside one of his six Tim Hortons establishments, mopping his forehead with a handkerchief. With a discerning look, he had assessed the two friends.

Simon said, "are you able to start training tomorrow"

"Absolutely," Alex replied without missing a beat, exchanging a glance with Mark, who gave an eager nod.

The following day, Alex and Mark stepped into the air-conditioned relief of Simon's Tim Hortons, ready for their first training session. Under the guidance of seasoned staff, they learned the ropes—brewing coffee, serving customers, managing inventory—all with the meticulous care of pharmacists dispensed to brewing the perfect cup. They absorbed every detail, every policy, every rhythm of the restaurant's pulse.

Two weeks of training flew by in a whirlwind of activity, and before they knew it, Alex and Mark found themselves donning crisp uniforms, name tags gleaming as they clocked in for their first official shift together, side by side, they worked the counters, filled orders, and navigated the ebb and flow of hungry patrons with precision.

"See that?" Alex whispered to Mark during a lull, gesturing towards their seamless teamwork. "Efficiency is our stepping stone to wealth."

Mark grinned, wiping down the counter. "One coffee at a time, my friend. One coffee at a time."

The Toronto sun blazed down unforgivingly, as Alex wiped his brow, feeling the sweat mingle with the determination set deep within him. Beside him, Mark squinted against the glare, both their gazes fixed on the Tim Hortons across the street where opportunity awaited in the guise of Simon, the owner of this and five other franchises in the bustling city.

"Ready for this?" Mark murmured, his voice steady despite the flutter of nerves that Alex knew danced in his friend's chest.

"Let's make it happen," Alex replied, his English clear and confident—a tool they'd both honed back home, unaware of how vital it would become in this new chapter of their lives.

The pair toiled, familiarizing themselves with the ins and outs of service, the rush of the morning crowd, and the lull in the afternoon. They learned to move in tandem, an efficient duo amidst the steam of coffee machines and the scent of freshly baked doughnuts. Their shifts started punctually at 8 am, ending at 4 pm—an eight-hour stretch where they poured every ounce of their ambition into each customer interaction.

A month passed, and the fruits of their labor began to manifest in the form of hard-earned Canadian dollars, the first seeds of their dream to cultivate wealth within a decade. It was during one of those routine evenings, the after-work glow still fresh on their faces, that Mark turned to Alex with a proposition that carried the weight of their shared aspirations.

"Alex, we're on the right path, but we've got to do more than just work," Mark said, the gym's fluorescent lights reflecting off his earnest expression. "We need to prime ourselves, body and mind. Set our alarms for 5 am, hit the gym, then tackle the day head-on."

Alex nodded, the idea resonating with him immediately. A healthy routine was the scaffolding upon which they could build their dreams—discipline in all things.

"Let's do it," he agreed, already visualizing the dark, pre-dawn mornings, the hum of the subway as they traveled post-workout, muscles tired but spirits unyielded. This was more than a job or a fitness regime; it was a testament to their resolve. They were pharmacists by trade, but now they were builders too—architects of their future, laying down the foundations for prosperity, one brick, one shift, one rep at a time.

Sweat beaded on Alex's forehead as he completed another set of deadlifts, the weight of the bar bending to his will. He glanced over at Mark, who was powering through a circuit of push-ups and pull-ups with a quiet intensity. The clank of metal and the muted thuds of rubber mats were a symphony to their new routine—these early morning sessions had become as integral to their day as the first sip of coffee.

"Alright," Mark panted, taking a brief respite on the bench beside Alex. "Next up: refueling. You remember what that nutritionist said?"

"Protein is king," Alex replied, toweling off his neck. "Builds muscle, repairs fibers... it's basically the currency our bodies trade in after a workout like this."

They made their way to the locker room, their muscles thrumming with exertion. They had learned quickly that discipline didn't stop at the gym doors; it threaded through every choice they made, weaving a tapestry of habits that would lead them to prosperity.

Showered and changed, they headed to a nearby market known for its fresh, organic produce. Rows upon rows of vibrant fruits and vegetables greeted them, but they moved purposefully toward the back where the butchers displayed their prime cuts of meat.

"Chicken breasts, salmon fillets, a dozen eggs," Mark recited from the list they'd compiled the night before. "Lean, mean protein machines."

"Let's grab some quinoa and black beans too," Alex suggested, eyeing the bulk bins. "Plant-based gains to mix things up."

Mark nodded in approval. There was a meticulousness to their approach now—every meal calculated; every calorie accounted for. They knew that the building blocks of their bodies' transformation were also the foundations of their dreams.

"Never thought I'd get excited about tuna and cottage cheese," Alex mused as they queued up at the checkout. His stomach growled in anticipation, craving the fuel that would sustain him through the afternoon shift.

"Hey, it's the small victories," Mark said, grinning. "Today it's tuna; tomorrow it's caviar."

Alex chuckled, imagining the opulent future they were constructing one rep, one meal, one disciplined step at a time. As they loaded their groceries into their backpacks, their conversation turned to recipes, to the subtle art of seasoning and marinating, to the shared joy of transforming raw ingredients into nourishment.

Leaving the market, they felt a sense of accomplishment that surpassed any physical exhaustion. This was more than a mere lifestyle change—it was a pledge, a commitment to embrace every aspect of the journey toward wealth. With each healthy choice, they were not only sculpting their bodies but also fortifying their resolve for the long road ahead.

The morning sun had barely begun to paint the Toronto skyline with hues of orange and pink when Alex's alarm pierced through the silence of his sparsely furnished apartment. Groaning, he slapped at the snooze button, only for a firm hand to grip his shoulder.

"Come on, Alex. Discipline, remember?" Mark's voice was both a grumble and encouragement, his silhouette outlined by the dawn light filtering in through the thin curtains.

Rubbing sleep from his eyes, Alex sat up, the weight of their ambition settling on his shoulders. Their pact to be rich within a decade wasn't just about money; it was a testament to their resolve, a challenge they had set for themselves in this new country that both intimidated and excited them.

"Alright, I'm up," Alex muttered, throwing off his covers. The cool air of the Canadian morning made him shiver as he dressed in workout gear, but the thought of warm coffee brewing at Tim Hortons spurred him on.

They arrived at the gym as the city was coming to life, the streets buzzing with early risers and the promise of a scorching summer day. The gym was quiet, save for the clanking of weights and the rhythmic thud of treadmills. Alex found solace in the routine, the steady burn in his muscles grounding him amidst the chaos of immigration and new beginnings.

"Feels good, doesn't it?" Mark said between sets, a bead of sweat trailing down his temple. "Keeping the body strong keeps the mind sharp."

"Agreed," Alex responded, pushing through another rep. They were pharmacists by education, but Simon's offer to work at one of his six bustling Tim Hortons locations had been an unexpected lifeline. They were quick learners, and after two weeks of training, they had fallen into the rhythm of their new roles with ease.

"Remember, man, it's not just about serving coffee and donuts," Mark would often remind him. "Every customer, every shift, it's a step closer to where we want to be."

Alex knew Mark was right. Each 8-hour shift from 8 am to 4 pm was an exercise in discipline, a trait they both acknowledged was crucial to climbing the ladder of success. As they wiped down the machines and headed for the showers, a silent agreement passed between them. This was more than a daily routine; it was the foundation upon which they'd build their dreams.

Exiting the gym, they felt the heat of the day beginning to assert itself, a stark contrast to the cool respite of the gym's air-conditioned interior. The walk to the subway station was short, and the ride gave them time to mentally prepare for the day ahead. It wasn't just about earning money; it was about learning, about growing, about forging their path in a land that offered opportunity at every turn.

"Today's going to be a good day," Mark said confidently, his breath fogging up the subway car's window.

Alex nodded, the train's rhythmic motion lulling him into a state of readiness. "Today, and every day after," he added, knowing full well the power of discipline to transform even the most ambitious of dreams into reality.

Sweat clung to Mark's brow as he hoisted the final rep of his deadlift, muscles taut and burning with exertion. Beside him, Alex racked his weights, a sense of accomplishment radiating from his tired frame. The clang of metal and the hum of treadmills surrounded them in a symphony of effort and endurance. They had committed themselves to this regimen, knowing their physical health was as crucial to their success as any job they worked.

"Protein shake?" Alex suggested, his voice steady despite the fatigue.

"Definitely," Mark replied, wiping his face with a towel. "We've got to fuel these gains if we're going to keep up with the pace we've set."

They made their way to the gym's cafe, where blenders whirred, and the smell of fresh fruit and nuts filled the air. Mark ordered two shakes, one with extra whey protein, while Alex surveyed the menu's healthy options. It wasn't just about building muscle; it was about nurturing their bodies to sustain the energy they needed to chase their dreams.

"Balance is key," Alex mused, accepting his shake. "Can't work or think straight if you're not taking care of the engine, right?"

"Exactly," Mark agreed, taking a long gulp of his shake, feeling the cool liquid course through him, replenishing what the workout had depleted. "And speaking of balance, I've been thinking about our plan. We can't leave anything to chance."

Alex nodded, curiosity piqued as they found a table and sat down, the cafe's chatter a backdrop to their more serious conversation.

"Here's what I'm proposing," Mark continued, pulling a small notebook from his gym bag. He opened it to a blank page, the paper crisp and unmarred. "We need structure, a roadmap for the next twelve months. Everything we do should be aimed toward our goal—being rich in ten years. Every decision, every sacrifice—it all needs to be documented."

"Write down every step..." Alex echoed thoughtfully, watching as Mark uncapped his pen with a decisive click. "It'll keep us honest, keep us moving forward."

"Right. So, month by month, we outline our objectives: savings targets, career milestones, networking opportunities, any side hustle ideas... everything." Mark's hand hovered above the paper, ready to etch their future into existence.

"Let's start with our current jobs, the gym routine, then look at certifications or further education. We could even explore investments, stocks, real estate..." Alex's voice trailed off, already envisioning the breadth of possibilities.

"Exactly. It'll evolve, but we need this foundation." Mark began to write, each word a commitment to their shared vision.

"Discipline in action," Alex said with a smile, raising his shake in a silent toast to the plan unfolding before them.

"Discipline in action," Mark affirmed, the scratch of pen on paper the sound of their ambitions taking form. With the blueprint of their future slowly filling the page, the two friends understood that wealth was not just about the money they would earn but the meticulous crafting of the life they intended to build.

The early morning sun filtered through the crowded skyline of Toronto as Alex and Mark emerged from the subway station, their conversations punctuated by the rhythmic clank of trains and the buzz of the city coming to life. They walked side by side, matching each other's stride with a synchronicity born from shared ambition.

"Mark," Alex said, his voice steady despite the thrumming energy of the city around them, "we've got our routine down, we're setting our foundation. But let's face it—as pharmacists working shifts at Tim Hortons, we'll make a living, not a fortune."

Mark nodded, the corner of his mouth quirking up in agreement as they sidestepped a group of hurried commuters.

"Agreed. So, what's the play?" he asked, his eyes meeting Alex's.

Alex took a deep breath, feeling the weight of their shared dream solidifying into resolve.

"We open our own businesses. That's how we build wealth, not just earn wages."

"Right, but we need to be recognized as pharmacists here first," Mark pointed out, a note of practicality threading through his excitement.

"Exactly. Which means understanding the Canadian requirements for our degrees," Alex continued, his mind already racing ahead to the challenges and possibilities that lay before them.

They reached the entrance to Simon's restaurant, the familiar aroma of coffee and baked goods greeting them like an old friend. Pausing before they stepped inside, Alex looked at Mark, his eyes alight with determination.

"Let's commit to this, Mark. Let's research every step of that process—what exams we need to pass, which credentials we must obtain, how much it will cost, everything. We'll add it to our plan."

"Consider it done," Mark replied, his hand on the door handle. "This is more than a job, Alex. This is about creating the lives we want."

With a mutual nod, they entered the establishment, ready to serve the day's first customers, but with minds firmly fixed on the future where they were not just employees, but entrepreneurs, masters of their own fate.

As the morning rush began to swell, Alex felt the familiar rhythm of work take hold. Between filling orders and managing inventory, his thoughts were never far from their goal. He watched Mark deftly handle the cash register, upselling a customer on a box of Timbits with a genuine smile.

"Discipline," Alex muttered under his breath, remembering Mark's earlier declaration. He knew that was the cornerstone of their success. It wasn't about grand gestures or sudden windfalls—it was about the daily grind, the incremental steps forward, the unwavering commitment to their plan.

"Hey, Alex," Mark called out during a lull, wiping down the counter. "After our shift, let's head straight to the library. We can start digging into the accreditation process."

"Good idea," Alex replied, tossing a used napkin into the trash. "The sooner we figure it out, the better."

They worked in tandem, a well-oiled machine born of two weeks' training and a decade-long friendship. As they clocked out at four, fatigue set in, but so did a sense of accomplishment. They had served hundreds of customers, saved more money towards their dreams, and were one step closer to understanding the path to their pharmacy degrees in Canada.

On the subway ride to the gym, Alex leaned against the window, watching the city blur by. Toronto was vast, diverse, and full of opportunity. It was also unforgiving, demanding resilience and hard work from those who sought to make it their home.

"Remember why we're doing this," Mark said, breaking into his reverie as they stepped off the train and headed towards the gym.

"Every push-up, every mile on the treadmill, it's not just about fitness. It's about proving to ourselves that we can stick to something—even when it's tough," Alex added, feeling a surge of energy despite the long day.

"Exactly. Discipline in the gym translates to discipline in life. And that's how we'll win," Mark concluded, pushing open the doors to the gym with a renewed vigor.

As they began their workout routine, Alex couldn't help but feel grateful for his friend's unwavering support and shared ambition. Together, they were more than just pharmacists from another country; they were dreamers forging a new future. And with each passing day, with every bead of sweat and every saved dollar, their ten-year goal didn't just seem possible—it felt inevitable.

The evening sun cast a warm glow through the window of their modest apartment as Alex and Mark huddled over a myriad of paperwork scattered across the kitchen table. Alex's brow furrowed in concentration, his fingers tracing lines of text in a thick reference book about Canadian pharmacy regulations.

"Mark," he said, pausing to glance up at his friend, "we've come a long way, but working these shifts isn't going to cut it if we're serious about making it big. We're pharmacists, sure, but here, we're just employees." He tapped the book with finality. "If we want wealth, real wealth, we need our own business. And that starts with getting our degrees recognized."

Mark nodded, his gaze fixed on a pamphlet titled 'International Pharmacy Graduates - Pathway to Licensure.' "I hear you, Alex. It's like we're stuck on this one rung of the ladder. We can't climb if we don't have the right credentials."

"Exactly." Alex leaned back, crossing his arms. "So, let's figure out what hoops we need to jump through to get our bachelor's degrees qualified here. Then we hit the books hard."

"Agreed. Tomorrow I'll make some calls, talk to the National Association of Pharmacy Regulatory Authorities, get the details." Mark scribbled a note in their shared planner, sliding it across to Alex for approval.

"Good. We'll divide and conquer," Alex said with a firm nod, feeling a surge of purpose. They were charting unknown territory, but together, they had always been an unstoppable force.

The next day unfolded in a flurry of phone calls, each one a step closer to clarity. They learned about exams, additional training, language proficiency tests—even the daunting task of securing internships. But by the end of the week, they had a clear picture of what needed to be done.

"Five months," Mark said, circling the date on the calendar. "That's when we sit for the evaluating exam. It gives us enough time to study without rushing."

"Five months," Alex repeated, his voice steady with resolve. They were pharmacists by trade, but now they were students once more, their evenings transformed into study sessions. Textbooks replaced TV shows, practice exams took the place of late-night outings. Each question answered was another brick laid on the foundation of their future empire.

As January approached, their routine was unyielding. Wake at dawn, hit the gym, work their shift, then study late into the night. Their eyes grew tired, but their spirits never wavered. They quizzed each other while preparing meals, discussed pharmacological interactions as they rode the subway, and challenged each other with complex cases they might encounter on the exam.

"Remember," Alex said during one of their study marathons, "this is just the beginning. The degree is the key that unlocks the door."

"And discipline," Mark added, tapping his temple, "is what will push that door wide open."

"Discipline and determination," Alex affirmed, a small smile creeping onto his face as he pictured the life that awaited them, just beyond the horizon of their ten-year plan.

Sweat dripped from Mark's brow as he counted the final, grueling repetitions of his early morning workout. Beside him, Alex grunted through his set, muscles straining, both pushing their bodies to the limit. The clang of weights and the rhythmic whir of treadmills surrounded them in the gymnasium that had become their temple of transformation.

"Protein shake?" Alex panted, wiping his forehead with a towel as they made their way to the cafe section of the gym.

"Double scoop," Mark replied, catching his breath. They needed the fuel, a concoction of nutrients to repair and build the muscle they had just broken down. It was about more than just getting fit; it was about conditioning themselves for the marathon ahead. Their regimen now included a strict diet - lean meats, legumes, and eggs were staples. Every meal was calculated for maximum energy and recovery. No more sugary indulgences or fast-food shortcuts. Their bodies were investments, and they treated them as such.

Later, sitting across from each other at a small table, notebooks open before them, they planned their future with the precision of pharmacists dispensing medicine.

"Okay, we'll start with the basics," Mark said, pen poised above the paper. "We save a portion of every paycheck. No exceptions."

"Right," Alex nodded in agreement, making a note. "And networking - we need to meet people who can mentor us, give us advice."

"Absolutely." Mark scribbled furiously. "Courses, certifications, whatever we need to advance. And let's not forget personal development. Books, seminars..."

"Health," Alex added, looking up from his notes. "We keep this routine. Gym five days a week, no excuses."

"Done." Mark underlined the commitment on the page. "This is our roadmap for the next year. We follow it to the letter."

"Every single day," Alex affirmed, his eyes reflecting the steel in his voice.

They reviewed their list: savings, networking, education, health. Each item was a step on the ladder to wealth, each action a brick in the fortress they were building. Discipline was their mortar, holding it all together. As they finalized their plan, their vision expanded beyond the confines of their current reality into a future where they weren't just surviving but thriving.

"Think of this as our declaration of independence," Mark said, a determined glint in his eye. "By this time next year, we'll be closer to our goal. We'll be unstoppable."

"Unstoppable," Alex echoed, the word tasting of promise and power.

They folded their plans, tucking them into their bags alongside their work uniforms and study materials. Stepping out into the crisp morning air, the city around them awakened to the possibilities of a new day, just as they had. With each sunrise, their resolve grew stronger, their dreams more vivid. And with their meticulously crafted plan etched in ink, the path to riches felt less like a distant dream and more like an inevitable destination.

The aroma of freshly ground coffee mingled with the scent of ambition as Alex and Mark sat at a corner table, their Tim Hortons uniforms folded neatly beside them. A laptop lay open, its screen awash with the glow of opportunity. Alex's fingers danced over the keyboard, navigating through web pages filled with information on Canadian equivalency standards for their pharmacy degrees.

"Mark," Alex said, glancing up from the screen. "We've been dispensing medications, but we're not really mixing our own success, are we? We can't just be employees forever."

Mark leaned in, his eyes scanning the criteria required for their degrees to be recognized in Canada. He nodded, his mind already calculating the steps ahead. "You're right, Alex. It's time we concoct our own formula for success. Let's start by understanding these qualification processes."

They discovered that they needed to pass an equivalency exam, a crucial step towards licensing. The task was daunting, yet it was a challenge they were willing to meet head-on, a pivotal move towards their goal of financial independence.

"Look here," Alex pointed at the screen, where the schedule for the Pharmacy Examining Board of Canada's assessment was displayed.

"Our study marathon begins now if we want to sit for this exam in January."

"Five months," Mark murmured, his brain already flipping through mental flashcards, pharmacology terms, and medical legislation. "That's our window. Let's break it down into daily goals."

"Daily goals, weekly check-ins," Alex suggested, closing the laptop with determination. They had their plan, their clue to navigate the labyrinth of regulations ahead.

"Alright, let's get started." Alex's voice held a resolute tone as he reached for a heavy pharmacology textbook. He flipped it open, the pages fluttering like the wings of their aspirations taking flight.

"Every page we turn, every chapter we digest," Mark added firmly, "brings us closer to the wealth we're after."

Together, they delved into the dense material, absorbing knowledge as they had absorbed protein in their disciplined diet. Their eyes were alight with focus, their minds sharp and eager. This was more than studying; it was the blueprint of their future fortunes, the very essence of their dreams distilled into the text before them.

"Here's to being rich in knowledge first," Alex toasted, raising his highlighter as though it were a glass of champagne.

"Then rich in life," Mark concluded, clinking his pen against Alex's marker.

They laughed softly, their shared vision binding them together stronger than any business contract ever could. They were more than friends; they were partners on a journey to prosperity, and the road ahead was clear.

Evening light spilled onto the table cluttered with textbooks, notepads brimming with scribbled notes, and a shared laptop open to a complex diagram of biochemical pathways. The faint hum of the city awakening outside their small apartment mingled with the sound of pages turning rapidly. Alex rubbed his eyes, weary yet wired from the relentless pursuit of their dream.

"Pharmacokinetics," he muttered under his breath, etching the term into his memory as he traced the curve of a graph showing drug absorption.

"Got it," Mark replied without looking up, his finger running down a column in his notebook. "Now onto pharmacodynamics."

They had divided the syllabus between them, each tackling different sections before teaching the other, solidifying their grasp on every concept. Their study sessions were marathons of dedication, fueled by the belief that each formula memorized, each drug interaction understood, brought them one step closer to their decade-long goal of wealth.

"Remember, it's about the receptors and the response," Alex said, distilling the information into manageable pieces.

"Right, the lock and key model," Mark chimed in, demonstrating with his hands. "Drug binds to receptor, effect occurs."

Their routine was set in stone: wake, gym, work, study. They moved through each day with a precision that mirrored the accuracy required in their field. Meals were brief, nutritious affairs; conversations revolved around aspirations and strategies.

"Let's drill side effects tomorrow morning," Alex proposed, marking a chapter with a sticky note. "It's crucial for the clinical section."

"Agreed," Mark nodded, his gaze never leaving the text. "And let's review contraindications too."

The room was a cocoon of concentration where time seemed to bend to their will. As the sky shifted from the pale blue of dawn to the deep azure of noon, they remained undeterred, their commitment unwavering.

"Think of it, Alex," Mark spoke up after a long silence, his voice steady with conviction. "Our own pharmacy, our name above the door..."

"Mark & Alex's," Alex mused, allowing himself a rare smile. "I like the sound of that."

"Me too," Mark agreed, returning the smile before they both dove back into the sea of medical jargon and treatment guidelines.

They were a unit, synchronized in purpose, their sights set firmly on the future. Every correct answer on their flashcards felt like a coin in their piggy bank of ambition. Each breakthrough in understanding was another brick laid on the path to their empire.

"Alright, break time's over," Alex declared after a moment, stretching his stiff muscles. "Let's go over those drug interactions again."

"Lead the way," Mark responded, just as eager to resume their journey through the thicket of knowledge.

They were pharmacists, yes, but more importantly, they were visionaries crafting their destiny with every studied word. Every single day spent in relentless preparation was a testament to their determination to reach the first step of their goal.

The first glimmers of dawn had yet to pierce the horizon when Alex's alarm pierced the silence of his small apartment. With a groan, he slapped at the snooze button but stopped himself midway, the weight of his ambitions heavy on his chest. He swung his legs off the bed with a determination that defied the early hour.

"Discipline," he muttered to himself, echoing the mantra that had become the foundation of his and Mark's shared dream. The word was a talisman, warding off the temptation of comfort and complacency.

He padded quietly to the cramped corner that served as their makeshift study area. Strewn across the desk were pharmacology texts they'd acquired second-hand, dog-eared notebooks filled with meticulous notes, and a calendar with dates crossed off leading to the middle of January. It wasn't much, but it was the launching pad for their future success.

Mark was already there, dark circles under his eyes betraying the late hours spent poring over the material. Yet, his focus was unbroken as he recited drug interactions from memory, a practice they'd adopted to ensure retention.

"Morning," Alex whispered, not wanting to break the sacred silence of their prep time.

"Morning," Mark replied, just as quietly, his finger following a line in one of the textbooks. "Let's get started."

They settled into a rhythm, the soft rustling of pages blending with the occasional murmur of recitation. There was no need for further conversation; both knew what was at stake.

Alex felt his brain absorbing information, transforming it into the knowledge that would be the cornerstone of their future business. It was a grind, the relentless repetition, the constant testing of each other, but it was also a forge, hardening their resolve and their friendship.

As the sky outside gradually lightened, signaling the approach of another day at Tim

Hortons, Alex couldn't help but feel a surge of pride. They were not only working towards their Canadian qualifications but also towards reshaping their destinies.

"Pharmacists today, proprietors tomorrow," Alex said softly to himself, an affirmation of the path they had chosen. Mark nodded without looking up, the agreement silent but absolute between them.

Their dedication was unwavering, each day carving a step closer to the summit of their aspirations. And with every correct answer, every concept mastered, the dream of wealth— of autonomy and success—felt less like a distant mirage and more like an impending reality.

Weeks swept by with the same disciplined rigor, the two friends relentlessly chasing dawn with a cocktail of protein shakes and pharmacology. The gym had become their sanctuary outside of work and study, a place where they could channel any lingering stress into the clank and heft of weights.

One particularly grueling morning, as they finished a punishing set of deadlifts, Mark's attention was captured by a pair of familiar faces across the room. They were there every morning, just like them—two women whose dedication to fitness rivaled their own. He nudged Alex, jerking his head subtly in their direction.

"Consistency," Alex noted, wiping the sweat from his brow with a towel. "The cornerstone of any success."

"Exactly," Mark agreed, his gaze lingering on the women who were now performing synchronized lunges. "And maybe it's about time we introduce ourselves, broaden our... network."

"Part of the plan?" Alex asked with a wry smile, though he couldn't deny his own curiosity about the two gym regulars.

"Networking is key in business and life," Mark quipped back, confirming his intentions without saying it outright.

With an unspoken agreement, they timed their water break to coincide with that of the women. Stepping over to the fountain, Mark initiated the conversation with a natural ease borne of genuine interest.

"Hey, I've noticed you're both as committed to your morning workouts as we are," he said, smiling warmly. "I'm Mark, and this is Alex."

"Hi," one of the women replied, her ponytail bouncing as she turned to face them. "I'm Sarah, and this is Emily. You guys are here early every day too, huh?"

"Every day without fail," Alex chimed in, offering a friendly nod. "It's part of our ten-year plan."

"Ten-year plan?" Emily asked, evidently intrigued.

"Yep," Mark jumped in, his enthusiasm clear. "We're pharmacists by trade, but we're studying for our Canadian qualifications. We're determined to be running our own business in a decade."

"Wow, that's ambitious," Sarah said, admiration flickering in her eyes.

"Life's too short for small dreams," Alex added, meeting Sarah's gaze with a steady one of his own.

The conversation flowed easily from there, the four of them finding common ground in their shared ambition and discipline. As they chatted, Alex felt a spark of connection, a sense of kinship that extended beyond the walls of the gym. It was refreshing to meet others who understood the value of hard work and clear goals.

As they parted ways, promising to catch up again during future workouts, Alex felt a renewed vigor. Yes, their journey towards wealth was still in its infancy, but moments like these reminded him that the path was not just about the destination; it was also about the relationships forged along the way.

"Seems like we've made more than just muscle gains today," Alex commented to Mark as they left the gym, the morning's encounter leaving a pleasant warmth in the wake of the usual post-workout exhaustion.

"Indeed," Mark agreed, his tone optimistic. "Who knows? Maybe our ten-year plan will include some unexpected partnerships."

"Or at least some friendly faces to share the grind with," Alex added, already looking forward to the next encounter, to the next opportunity, to the next step toward their goal.

"Exactly," Mark said, a thoughtful look crossing his features. "You know, Alex, these connections could be the extra push we need. A little competition, some camaraderie—it's motivating."

Alex nodded, feeling the weight of their shared dreams propelling him forward. As they strode towards the subway station, he replayed the morning's interaction, analyzing Sarah and Emily's responses, the way their eyes lit up when talking about their own aspirations. It was invigorating to meet people who didn't just talk but acted on their ambitions.

"Plus, it's nice to have someone else to talk to about all this," Alex admitted, thinking out loud. "We've been in our bubble—study, work, gym. It's easy to get tunnel vision."

"True," Mark responded, his voice echoing in the hollow subway corridor. "Balance is key. We're here to build a life, not just a bank account."

The train arrived with a rush of air, its doors sliding open to welcome them. They stepped inside, finding seats amidst the early morning commuters. Alex pulled out a small notebook from his bag—a habit he had developed to jot down thoughts and observations throughout the day.

"Tonight," Alex said, flipping open to a blank page, "let's review our progress. Adjust the plan if needed. And maybe pencil in some time for socializing. It's about discipline, yes, but also about enjoying the journey."

"Agreed," Mark said, leaning back against the seat. "Let's keep moving forward, without losing sight of the world around us."

As the train glided through the tunnels, whisking them towards another day of striving toward their dreams, Alex felt a sense of contentment. Yes, the road ahead was long and undoubtedly filled with challenges, but as long as they remained focused and open to the world's surprises, the future was bright. With determination, discipline, and now new friendships blossoming, Alex knew that their ten-year plan was more than just a dream—it was a blueprint for success.

The gym was bustling with the clanks and grunts of morning exertion when Alex spotted Sarah and Emily on the treadmills. He nudged Mark, who was re-racking his weights, and nodded in their direction.

"Let's do it now, before we lose our nerve," Alex whispered, feeling a flutter of anticipation in his stomach.

Mark wiped the sweat from his brow and straightened up, his posture exuding the confidence that Alex sometimes envied. Together, they approached the two women, who were now stretching as cool down from their run.

"Hey, Sarah, Emily," Mark started, his tone casual yet clear over the hum of activity. "How's the workout going?"

"Good!" Sarah replied with a smile, her ponytail bobbing. "You guys seem to be killing it as usual."

"Trying to keep up with you," Alex chimed in, earning a light laugh from Emily.

"Actually," Mark said, shifting slightly, "we were wondering if you'd like to grab a coffee with us sometime? Outside the gym, I mean."

Alex held his breath, aware of the stakes. They had talked about the importance of building relationships, of networking beyond the confines of work and study. This was part of their plan—expanding their circle, exploring opportunities, learning from others.

"Sounds nice," Emily responded, sharing a glance with Sarah. "We could use a break from protein shakes and energy bars."

"Great! How about tomorrow after our workout?" Alex suggested, feeling a surge of relief.

"Perfect," Sarah agreed. "There's a nice café just a couple of blocks from here."

"Tomorrow it is," Mark confirmed with a nod, pleased with the outcome.

They exchanged goodbyes and went back to their routines, but Alex noted a new buoyancy in their steps. As he pumped through his last set of reps, his mind wasn't only on the weight he was lifting but also on the possibilities that lay ahead. Yes, they were in Canada to build a future, a financially secure life, but along the way, they would forge connections that could prove its valuable

"Discipline and planning," Alex reminded himself silently, already looking forward to tomorrow's coffee. "But never forget to live in the moment."

The anticipation of the coffee date with Sarah and Emily buzzed through Alex's mind like caffeine through his veins. He lay in bed, the neon glow of a streetlight outside casting a dim light across the ceiling of the apartment he shared with Mark. Sleep was a distant dream, chased away by the thrill of new connections and the potential they represented.

"Mark," he whispered across the room, where his friend's form lay motionless under the covers. There was no response. "You awake?"

A muffled groan answered him. "Now I am."

"Sorry," Alex said sheepishly, "I just can't sleep. Excited about tomorrow, you know?"

"Tell me about it," Mark muttered, sitting up. "Our first real non-work-related outing since we got here. Feels like a step towards something bigger, doesn't it?"

"Exactly." Alex sat up too, propping himself against the headboard. "It's not just about meeting Sarah and Emily. It's about building our life here, making the most of every opportunity."

"Part of the ten-year plan," Mark added, a note of determination cutting through the haze of sleep. "Remember, discipline."

"Discipline," Alex echoed. "But also enjoying the journey. Balancing the grind with moments like these."

"Speaking of balance, we took off work for this. Simon will expect us to make up for it,"

Mark reminded him, his voice now fully awake.

"True, but we've been solid employees. He knows he can count on us." Alex's confidence wasn't just bravado; their work ethic had already made a good impression on Simon.

"Alright then," Mark said, a touch of excitement creeping into his voice. "Let's try to get some rest. Big day tomorrow."

"Goodnight, Mark."

"Goodnight, Alex."

They settled back into their beds, the silence returning to the room. Despite their lack of sleep, there was a shared understanding that moments like the one awaiting them were rare gems to be cherished—opportunities for laughter, learning, and perhaps the spark of an idea that could lead to the wealth they sought. With the promise of tomorrow fueling their dreams, Alex and Mark finally drifted off to sleep, the blueprint of their future silently etching itself into the night.

The rising sun poured its light through the blinds, casting luminous streaks across the room as Alex's eyes blinked open. Beside him, Mark was already up, his bed made with military precision—a testament to their shared creed of discipline.

"Morning, champ," Mark greeted, his tone light but his eyes betraying a hint of anticipation for the day ahead.

"Morning," Alex replied, a smile tugging at the corners of his mouth. The excitement from last night resurfaced, igniting a spark in his chest. Today wasn't just about routines; it was about connections, about the potential woven into new friendships—or perhaps something more.

In sync, they donned their gym attire, a ritual that had become second nature. Their movements were brisk yet unhurried, each step a small victory in the march towards their dreams. As they exited their modest apartment, the crisp morning air greeted them, a silent ally in their quest for success.

The walk to the gym was short, but today it felt charged with possibility. They entered, nodding to familiar faces, but their focus was elsewhere, searching.

And there they were—Sarah and Emily, engaged in a lively discussion by the treadmills, their laughter echoing off the walls like a siren song. Alex and Mark exchanged a

glance, their smiles broadening. This was it—
the simple joy of connection that made all the
hard work worth it.

"Hey, guys!" Sarah called out, waving them
over. Emily's smile mirrored her friend's
warmth as they approached.

"Ready for that coffee?" Mark asked, his usual
confidence blending with a touch of nervous
energy.

"Absolutely," Emily responded, her eyes
sparkling with enthusiasm.

Together, the group stepped outside, the gym's
ambiance giving way to the bustling streets of
Toronto. The city was alive with the sounds of
progress, a symphony that spoke of endless
possibilities. Alex and Mark fell into step with
the girls, their conversation flowing as freely as
the pedestrians around them.

They reached the coffee shop—a quaint place
with an inviting aroma that promised rich
blends and sweet pastries. As they settled into
a cozy corner, the initial excitement melded
into comfortable camaraderie. This was more
than just a break from routine; it was a clue, a
reminder from the universe that while wealth

was their goal, the richness of life lay in moments like these.

"Cheers," Alex said, raising his cup in a toast to friendship, to dreams, and to the endless pursuit of happiness that defined their journey.

"Cheers," echoed Mark, Sarah, and Emily in unison, the clink of their cups a tangible affirmation of the new bonds forming around the small table.

As they sipped on their coffee, the conversation naturally meandered towards ambitions and aspirations. It was Alex who steered the dialogue to the heart of their shared dream.

"You know," he began, his voice a mix of earnestness and excitement, "Mark and I, we've got this plan. We want to be more than just pharmacists; we want to build something of our own."

Mark nodded, taking over with ease. "We're talking about discipline, determination. We hit the gym every morning, eat right, stay focused. It's all part of the bigger picture, you know?"

Sarah leaned forward, her interest piqued. "That sounds intense, but amazing. What's the ultimate goal?"

"To be rich in ten years," Alex admitted, not without some trepidation. "Not just money-wise, but rich in experiences, in achievements."

Emily's eyes reflected genuine admiration. "I love that. So many people just talk, but you both are actually doing something about it."

The exchange continued, each revelation about their rigorous routine and steadfast commitment to their goals drawing impressed nods from Sarah and Emily. Alex and Mark spoke with passion, detailing the steps they were taking to reach their ambitious target, how they balanced their jobs at Tim Hortons with studying for their degree qualifications, all while maintaining a strict regimen.

It was more than just a plan laid out on paper; it was a living, breathing journey that they were navigating with unwavering intent. And as they shared their story, their animated expressions and lively gestures conveyed the depth of their conviction.

"Wow," Sarah exclaimed, a hint of awe coloring her tone. "You guys really have it all figured out."

"It's not just about figuring it out," Mark said with a grin. "It's about following through. One step at a time, right, Alex?"

"Exactly," Alex agreed. "And today, well, meeting you two is definitely one of those good steps."

Laughter filled the space between them, light and easy, yet underscored by a shared understanding that there was something truly special unfolding. As the conversation drifted to lighter topics, the foundation of a deeper connection had been laid—a connection built on dreams, discipline, and the undeniable allure of a future crafted by their own hands.

Emily leaned forward, her eyes dancing with curiosity and respect. "It's inspiring to hear you talk about your plans. It's not every day you meet people who are so dedicated."

"Thank" you," Alex said, feeling a surge of pride. "But enough about us for now. What about you two? What brings you to the gym at the crack of dawn?"

"Survival," Sarah joked, then grew more serious. "We're in our third year of civil engineering at the university. It's demanding, and keeping fit helps us manage the stress."

"Plus, we have our own dreams of building something lasting," Emily added, her gaze steady and full of that same fiery determination that Alex recognized in himself and Mark. "Bridges, buildings... maybe even empires."

The conversation flowed effortlessly from there, each revelation about Sarah and Emily echoing Alex and Mark's drive for success. It wasn't just their shared dedication to discipline and ambition that resonated—it was the underlying belief that hard work could forge the path to their dreams.

As they spoke of late-night study sessions and complex projects, Alex saw a reflection of his and Mark's journey. The four of them were different pieces of the same puzzle, striving for greatness in their respective fields, yet bound by an unspoken kinship that only those who dare to chase lofty goals could truly understand.

"Sounds like you're as committed to your future as we are," Mark said, admiration clear in his voice.

"Absolutely," Sarah replied. "We have big plans, and we're sticking to them."

"Then it seems we have more in common than we thought," Alex concluded, the connection between them solidifying with each shared dream and laugh.

In this moment, surrounded by the hum of the coffee shop, the four young dreamers allowed themselves to bask in the warmth of newfound friendships and the recognition that they weren't alone in their quests for success.

"Engineering's a tough field," Mark continued, leaning forward, his enthusiasm palpable. "But I bet you both have what it takes to reshape the landscape of Prospera."

Emily smiled at the mention of their divided city, a spark in her eyes. "That's the plan. We want to design structures that bridge the gap between the upper tiers and lower slums, make life better for everyone."

"Admirable," Alex said earnestly. The idea resonated with him deeply, given the stark contrasts they had observed since arriving in Toronto. He saw potential in these young women, not just as engineers but as visionaries who could one day influence the fabric of society.

"And challenging," Sarah added, "given how technology is rapidly changing and the Empire keeps a tight grip on resources. But we believe in making a difference, no matter the obstacles."

"Much like us," Alex agreed, feeling a sense of camaraderie. "We're pharmacists by trade, but we know that staying employees won't get us where we need to be. That's why we're aiming high—our own business, our own way."

"Sounds like we all refuse to let the confines of our current circumstances dictate our futures," Emily remarked, her gaze meeting Alex's.

"Exactly," Mark chimed in. "And discipline will get us there. Just like your designs will need a strong foundation, our goals require a solid base of hard work and persistence."

As they talked, Alex noticed the way the girls' optimism mirrored his and Mark's ambitions. They were not deterred by the oppressive atmosphere of the lower tiers or the daunting silhouette of the Cyberspire. Instead, they were fueled by the challenges, driven to succeed despite—or perhaps because of—the hardships.

"Maybe one day, your buildings will stand tall among the skyscrapers," Alex suggested, gesturing through the window towards the distant skyline, "and our pharmacy will cater to those seeking healing, powered by faith and science alike."

The thought brought collective smiles to their faces, and for a moment, the weight of the journey ahead felt lighter. They were no longer just two sets of ambitious strangers; they were allies in aspiration, united in their pursuit of a future where dreams transformed into reality.

"Let's make a pact then," Sarah proposed, her eyes sparkling with the kind of enthusiasm that's infectious. "To stay positive, to keep each other motivated, no matter how tough it gets."

"Deal," Alex agreed without hesitation, his hand outstretched across the table.

Mark's hand followed, and then Emily's, their four hands coming together in a stack, a tangible representation of their shared commitment. It was more than a gesture; it was a silent vow, an unspoken understanding that they were now part of something larger than themselves.

"We'll help each other," Emily added, her voice steady with conviction. "Whether it's exam stress or business hurdles, we're in this together."

"Absolutely," Mark said. "We all have different skills to bring to the table, and that's our advantage."

They nodded in agreement, their hands disentangling as they sat back, the pact sealed. The conversation shifted naturally afterward, as they delved into lighter topics—favorite foods, music tastes, the odd laugh about gym quirks. But beneath the casual chatter, the promise lingered, binding them.

Hours passed without notice, the shadows lengthening as the sun began its descent behind the towering cityscape. It was time to part ways, but the farewell was not tinged with sadness. Instead, there was a sense of anticipation, a zest for what was to come.

"See you at the gym tomorrow?" Alex asked, hope threading through his words.

"Wouldn't miss it," Sarah smiled, while Emily nodded in agreement.

With a final round of goodbyes, Alex and Mark stepped out of the coffee shop, the bell above the door chiming a soft conclusion to their meeting. They walked side by side in comfortable silence, each man lost in thought.

"Sarah's incredible, isn't she?" Alex finally broke the silence, a grin spreading across his face.

"Emily's pretty amazing too," Mark responded, matching his friend's expression. "I think today was a good day—not just for our future plans, but... personally."

"Agreed," Alex replied. "Meeting them felt like... another piece of the puzzle falling into place."

As they reached the subway station, they couldn't help but feel that their steps were a little lighter, their spirits a little brighter. The journey ahead was still long and uncertain, but with newfound allies and mutual support, the path seemed less daunting.

"Ten years," Alex mused aloud, the train rumbling in the distance. "It doesn't seem so far away now."

"Ten years," Mark echoed, his gaze fixed on the horizon, where the last rays of sunlight kissed the edges of the world. "We'll get there, one step at a time."

The train ride home was a blur of motion and muffled sounds, but within their shared gaze, there was a clarity that spoke volumes. Side by side, they contemplated the day's events, each replaying the interactions with Sarah and Emily in their minds. The rhythmic clacking of the train seemed to synchronize with the steady beat of possibility in their chests.

Once home, they hung their jackets on the coat rack and slipped off their shoes, the familiarity of the apartment wrapping around them like an old friend. It was here, in this humble space, that their dreams were taking shape, fueled by discipline and now, a touch of serenity.

Alex flopped onto the couch, his head tipping back as he stared at the ceiling, lost in thought. "Sarah has this energy about her," he began, his voice tinged with admiration. "It's like she sees right through the mundane stuff and finds what's really worth focusing on."

Mark took a seat opposite him, nodding slowly. "Emily's got this quiet strength, you know? She listens... really listens. It makes you want to open up, share things you didn't even realize you were holding onto."

"Tomorrow," Alex said softly, a decisive edge to his tone, "we're getting those phone numbers."

"Absolutely," Mark agreed, the determination evident in his eyes. "It's not just about us anymore. It's about building something bigger, together—with them."

They sat in silence for a moment, the weight of their aspirations settling upon them, yet somehow lightened by the prospect of shared journeys. Tomorrow was more than just another day; it was another step toward their dream, enriched by new connections and potential.

"Ten years," Alex whispered into the quiet of the room, the phrase becoming their mantra.

"Ten years," Mark affirmed, and in his voice was the echo of every dreamer who had dared to reach beyond the horizon.

With that, they retired to their respective rooms, the image of Sarah and Emily etched into their thoughts. Sleep would come, but it would be restless, charged with anticipation for the dawn of a new day—a day when they would take yet another stride towards the future they envisioned.

The morning sun filtered through the blinds, casting a warm glow on Alex's face as he stirred awake. Today was charged with a new kind of energy. He rolled out of bed, his thoughts instantly gravitating towards Sarah—the way her laughter seemed to resonate with his own sense of humor, her ambitious glint mirroring his.

Mark was already up, the clatter of breakfast preparations drifting from the kitchen. They had a ritual—a protein-packed meal to fuel their grueling day ahead—and today was no exception. But amidst the routine, an undercurrent of excitement bubbled beneath the surface.

"Big day," Mark called out, flipping an omelet expertly in the pan.

"Could be a game-changer," Alex replied, splashing water on his face, awakening his senses fully.

They ate quickly, their conversation orbiting around the usual—work, gym, study plans—but there was a palpable buzz about what would come after: the simple act of asking for a phone number, yet so much hinged on it.

At the gym, they found their rhythm, the weights, and cardio machines a prelude to the real workout for their confidence. When Sarah and Emily arrived, cheerful and bright as the morning itself, Alex and Mark exchanged a glance; it was time.

"Hey, Sarah," Alex began, his heart drumming a rapid beat as he approached her after the session. She was wiping down her treadmill, ponytail swaying. "Would you, uh, mind if I got your number? Maybe we could grab a coffee outside of here sometime?"

Sarah's smile beamed, and there was no hesitation. "Sure, Alex. I'd like that," she said, punching her digits into his phone.

Meanwhile, Mark found Emily stretching by the free weights. "Emily, I was wondering..." He paused, collecting his thoughts. "Could I have your number? It'd be great to continue our chat from yesterday."

"Of" course, Mark," Emily responded warmly, extending her phone towards him. "I'm looking forward to it."

As Alex and Mark reconvened, they couldn't help but feel a surge of triumph. They had taken a step toward something meaningful—

not just with Sarah and Emily, but with their own reflections.

"See what I mean?" Alex said, his grin infectious. "They're driven, just like us. They have dreams, ambitions. It's like looking into a mirror and seeing a part of yourself staring back."

"Exactly," Mark agreed, his eyes alight with the acknowledgment of a shared understanding. "We came here to build a future, and now, maybe, we've found companions for the journey."

They left the gym, numbers secured in their phones, the promise of new beginnings interlaced with the pursuit of their goals. In Sarah and Emily, they recognized their own drive and determination, and it drew them closer. They were more than just potential romantic interests; they were allies in ambition, partners in the dream that Alex and Mark were determined to make a reality.

"Ten years," Alex murmured once again, a content smile on his lips.

"Ten years," Mark echoed, and together they stepped out into the bustling Toronto streets, their path illuminated by the clarity of their vision and the companionship they had found.

Sweat still glistened on their foreheads as Alex and Mark made their way through the throng of morning commuters, heading toward the subway station. The cool underground air was a welcome respite from the lingering heat of the workout.

"Man, that was a killer session," Mark said, adjusting the strap of his gym bag over his shoulder.

"Nothing we can't handle," Alex replied with a chuckle. "Gotta keep pushing if we're going to make it."

They descended the stairs to the subway platform, the familiar rumble of an approaching train vibrating beneath their feet. As they waited, Alex turned to Mark, his expression turning serious. "You know, even with Sarah and Emily in the picture now, we can't lose sight of why we're here."

Mark nodded, his gaze meeting Alex's. "Absolutely. They're incredible, but our dreams come first. We can't forget that. We're going to be rich, build our empire. That's the promise we made to each other."

"Exactly," Alex affirmed. "We've got a plan, and nothing's going to derail us—not even romance. We'll balance it all. Discipline, remember?"

"Discipline is key," Mark agreed, just as the train pulled into the station with a screech of brakes against metal. "And we're disciplined guys. That's how we'll succeed."

The doors slid open, and the pair stepped inside the crowded car, finding a spot where they could stand shoulder-to-shoulder amidst the sea of passengers. They held onto the overhead rails as the train lurched forward, carving its path beneath the city.

"First, we get our degrees recognized," Alex stated, his voice steady despite the jostling of the train. "Then, we start climbing. Pharmacy today, but tomorrow—who knows? Our own business, maybe multiple businesses. Investments. Real estate."

"Exactly," Mark said, a fire igniting in his eyes. "We'll stay grounded, work hard, study harder. We'll save every penny we earn at Tim Hortons, and we'll invest wisely. And sure, having girlfriends could be part of this new life, but they won't distract us from our goals."

"Sarah and Emily seem like the kind who would push us even further," Alex mused, a smile tugging at the corner of his mouth. "They understand ambition. Maybe together, we'll reach even greater heights."

"Partners in every sense," Mark said, as the train neared their stop. "Alright, let's head to work. We've got a long day ahead, and we need every hour we can get."

As the train slowed, the friends exchanged a look of solidarity. With every step, every shift at the restaurant, every page of their textbooks, they were building the foundation of their future—a future they were determined to shape with unwavering dedication, whether they walked the road alone or with someone special by their side.

The subway doors slid open with a hiss, disgorging Alex and Mark into the thrum of Toronto's morning rush. They surged forward with the crowd, their gym bags slung over their shoulders, muscles warmed from the early workout, minds sharpened for the day ahead.

"Remember that biochem section we were stuck on?" Mark asked as they navigated the throngs of commuters heading to work.

"Which one? There have been too many," Alex replied with a chuckle. "But yeah, I think we're getting the hang of it."

"Emily suggested that study group at the university library. We should join them next week," Mark suggested, adjusting the strap of his bag. "Sarah mentioned some useful resources there, too."

"Good idea," Alex agreed. "They've been through this already. It's like having our own personal guides through the maze of exams and certifications."

"Man, between Simon's training at Tim Hortons and the girls' help at the gym and studies... We're set up better than we thought."

"True," Alex nodded. "We've got a support system. And discipline—that's what will make us rich in ten years. Not just the money, but rich in knowledge, experience, and relationships."

"Exactly. Now let's get through today, so we can tackle tomorrow," Mark said as they stepped out of the station and into the daylight.

With the city bustling around them, they walked side by side towards the familiar red and brown hues of the Tim Hortons where they worked. Their shifts were demanding, but every order they filled, every customer they served, was another step toward their grand ambition. And when the day was done, they would return home to their shared apartment, their sanctuary of dreams and determination, where textbooks awaited to challenge their resolve.

Yet, no matter how exhausting the routine, Alex and Mark never wavered. They supported each other through every setback and celebrated every small victory because they knew each success brought them closer to the life they envisioned. They had made a pact to be rich in 10 years, and nothing—not even the sweet distraction of new relationships—could pull them astray from the path they had set for themselves.

The library's fluorescent lights hummed overhead, casting a sterile glow over the rows of books and study carrels. Alex and Mark settled into their usual spot with an air of quiet determination, textbooks and notebooks splayed before them like battle plans.

"Okay," Mark said as he cracked his knuckles, "pharmacology first, then onto biochemistry."

"Agreed," Alex replied, pulling out his color-coded flashcards. They had devised a system to tackle the dense material: summarize, quiz, review. It was a process that had served them well, translating into the language of persistence that they both spoke fluently.

Beside them, the girls, Sarah and Emily, were absorbed in their own studies, but the four had created a silent pact of mutual encouragement. The occasional glance, the shared nods of comprehension, and the whispered words of motivation tied them together in their common pursuit of excellence.

Hours ticked by, measured in page turns and scribbled notes. They dove deep into the complexities of human physiology, dissecting mechanisms of action and drug interactions with a fervor that would have impressed any professor. This wasn't just about passing exams; it was about mastering a craft, about laying the foundation for the businesses they aspired to build.

"Hey, check this out," Alex said at one point, breaking the silence. He pointed to a diagram explaining a particularly tricky concept. Mark leaned in, and together they unraveled the mystery, their minds syncing up in understanding.

"Got it," Mark said, a grin spreading across his face. "We're going to ace this exam."

"Without a doubt," Alex agreed, the fatigue of the day momentarily forgotten.

As midnight approached, they began to pack up their things, the library now nearly deserted. They stood and stretched, their bodies protesting the long hours of immobility.

"Same time tomorrow?" Sarah asked, her own stack of books in hand.

"Wouldn't miss it," Mark replied, while Alex nodded in agreement.

They left the library together, the night air crisp and invigorating. As they parted ways, Alex and Mark knew that the path they had chosen was not an easy one. But with each other—and now with Sarah and Emily by their sides—they felt invincible. They were more than just students or pharmacists; they were dreamers in pursuit of a future rich in every sense of the word.

And so, under the starlit sky of Toronto, they walked home, their spirits undimmed, ready to rise with the sun and do it all over again. Because every day spent studying hard was another step toward their ten-year goal—a goal that seemed less like a dream and more like an inevitability with every passing moment.

The frigid January winds whipped through the streets of Toronto as Alex and Mark, bundled in their winter coats, trudged toward their shared apartment. They could see their breath in the air, a misty indication of the effort that had gone into their day.

"Remember when we thought this would be just about memorizing drug interactions?" Alex joked, huffing out clouds of warm air.

Mark chuckled, "Yeah, if only. Pharmacology is one thing, but Canadian regulations are a whole different beast."

Their strides were purposeful, each step a testament to the resilience they had built over these past months. The exam was looming—a towering giant on the horizon of their aspirations. But they were ready. They had come too far, invested too much of themselves to falter now.

"Hey," Mark said suddenly, his voice taking on a serious tone. "You ever get that feeling like we're right on the edge of something big? Like all of this—" He gestured broadly, encompassing everything from the snow-lined streets to the endless nights of study, "—is about to pay off?"

"Every day," Alex replied, smiling despite the jitters that danced in his stomach. "We made a promise to ourselves. Ten years to make it big. We can't let a little—or a lot—of nerves stop us now."

They reached their apartment building, the familiar buzz of the entryway greeting them like an old friend. Stepping inside, they shrugged off the cold along with their jackets.

"Alright, last review session tonight?" Alex asked, already heading toward the kettle to brew some strong coffee for the long night ahead.

"Last one," confirmed Mark, pulling out stacks of flashcards they had created.

As the kettle whistled its readiness, the comforting aroma of coffee filled the small kitchen, acting as a soothing balm to their frazzled nerves. They settled at the table, mugs in hand, surrounded by books and notes that seemed to stretch on infinitely.

"Let's focus on the clinical case studies," Alex suggested. "They're likely to throw a few curveballs our way with those."

"Agreed," said Mark, flipping open a textbook to a particularly dense chapter.

Hours passed, their concentration unwavering despite the weight of sleeplessness bearing down upon them. They quizzed each other, debated treatment options, and clarified complex mechanisms of action until the words began to blur together.

"Okay, I think that's enough for tonight," Mark finally conceded as the early light of dawn began to filter through the blinds.

"Agreed," Alex said, his brain saturated with information, yet surprisingly clear. "We know this stuff, Mark. We really do."

"Absolutely," Mark nodded, confidence slowly overtaking the nervous energy that had fueled their marathon session.

They rose from the table, a silent pact between them that no more words were needed. Tomorrow, they would face the exam together—nervous, yes, but also without a shadow of a doubt about their capacity to succeed.

As they crawled into bed, the first hints of sunlight creeping into their room, they allowed themselves the brief luxury of imagining life after the exam. The future was bright, tangible, and within reach; it was just beyond the horizon of tomorrow's challenge.

And in their hearts, they knew—they would conquer it, just as they had conquered every obstacle before. Because they weren't just friends or pharmacists. They were Alex and Mark, two dreamers who had set out to turn their ambitions into reality, no matter what stood in their way.

The alarm blared at a merciless volume, but Alex and Mark were already stirring. With military precision, they rolled out of bed, their bodies conditioned by months of early gym sessions. The remnants of fatigue clung stubbornly to their limbs, but the spark of determination in their eyes burned it away.

"Let's do this," Alex said, his voice steady with resolve.

"Today's the day we've been working towards," Mark replied, matching Alex's unspoken intensity.

Breakfast was a quiet affair, each man lost in his own thoughts, mentally reviewing pharmacological processes and drug interactions. They dressed in comfortable clothing, the unofficial armor of test-takers, designed for endurance rather than style.

The journey to the exam center was a blur. They navigated the familiar streets of Toronto, now imprinted in their muscle memory from countless subway rides to work and the library. The city was just waking up, its rhythm syncing with their own anticipation.

Upon arrival, the exam center was already buzzing with the nervous energy of fellow candidates. Alex and Mark exchanged a glance, a silent communication that had become their secret language over the years. In that look was every late-night study session, every shared dream, every whispered encouragement when the weight of their ambition seemed too heavy.

"Remember, we're not just here to pass. We're here to excel," Mark murmured, his confidence infectious.

"Exactly," Alex replied, nodding. "We've put in the work. We know our stuff. Let's show them what we're made of."

With heads held high, they entered the exam room. The desks were neatly arranged in rows, each one a small island in a sea of potential. They found their assigned seats, the numbers on their admission slips corresponding to those on the desks.

As the invigilator called for silence and began to distribute the exam papers, Alex and Mark took a deep breath. This was it—the culmination of all their efforts, the gateway to the future they had envisioned so meticulously.

"Begin," the invigilator announced, and with a collective rustle of paper, the room fell into a hush.

Pens in hand, Alex and Mark dove into the questions, their minds razor-sharp, their focus unwavering. They worked methodically, confidently, as if the answers were a part of them, etched into their DNA.

And as the final minutes ticked away, they emerged from their concentration, looking up almost simultaneously. Their expressions mirrored each other—satisfied, relieved, victorious. They had done everything within their power, and now, their fate rested in the hands of time and grading.

But one thing was certain: they had walked into the exam center with full confidence, and they would walk out with it too. Because no matter the outcome, Alex and Mark knew they had already succeeded. They had turned strangers into friends, challenges into triumphs, and dreams into plans. And that was worth more than any test result.

With the invigilator's final call signaling the end of the grueling hours, Alex and Mark laid down their pens. They exchanged a glance that bounced with a mix of exhaustion and anticipation, nodding to each other as they began to collect their belongings.

"Let's step outside," Mark whispered, his voice a mixture of fatigue and the remnants of adrenaline from the last few hours of intense focus.

They shuffled through the corridors, their footsteps synchronizing with the heartbeat of their shared ambition. Once outside, they inhaled the crisp winter air, a welcome relief after the stifling atmosphere of determination and pencils scratching against paper.

"Time to make that call," Alex said, his finger hovering over his phone with hesitant excitement.

"Go for it," Mark encouraged, clapping him on the back as he watched his friend dial the number.

"Hey Sarah," he began, the receiver crackling slightly before her voice came through, warm and expectant.

"Hey! How did it go?" Sarah's voice bubbled with curiosity.

Mark watched as Alex paced a little, kicking at the snow that had accumulated at the edge of the sidewalk.

"We gave it our all," Alex replied, trying to keep his tone light, "but you never know with these things, right? We have to wait a month for the results."

"Emily and I are sure you guys nailed it," she reassured him, her confidence infectious even through the phone. "You've worked so hard."

"Thanks, we hope so," Alex responded, allowing himself a small smile. "We'll celebrate when we know for sure."

"Definitely! Call us as soon as you hear anything, okay?"

"Will do," Alex promised, ending the call.

He looked over at Mark, who was watching the exchange with an unreadable expression. "Your turn," Alex nudged, handing over the phone.

"Hey Emily," Mark started, his voice steady but with an undercurrent of nerves that hadn't quite settled yet. "It feels good to be done, but the real test is waiting for the results."

"Whatever happens, I'm proud of you both," Emily's clear voice came through, soothing like a balm to the anxious energy that still lingered around them. "You two are the most disciplined people I know."

"Thanks, Em," Mark said, a genuine smile breaking through. "That means a lot."

"Keep us updated, alright?" she said before bidding goodbye.

As they hung up, the weight of the moment seemed to settle on them. They stood side by side, taking in the silence that followed the storm of their efforts. Their dream—once a distant star on the horizon—now felt tangibly close, just within their reach. But for now, all they could do was wait.

"Come on," Mark finally said, breaking the quiet. "Let's head to work. Simon won't run those Tim Hortons by himself."

And with that, they started off toward the subway station, the familiar rhythm of their routine comforting in its predictability. They walked shoulder to shoulder, the bond of their friendship and shared aspirations an unspoken oath between them.

The night had draped Toronto in a blanket of stillness, the hustle of daytime replaced by the hushed whispers of the dark. Alex and Mark sat on the worn couch in their modest apartment, the dim glow from a single lamp casting long shadows across the room.

"Remember when we first got here?" Alex mused, his gaze lost somewhere in the past. "We thought just speaking English would make everything smooth sailing."

Mark chuckled softly. "Yeah"

"Turns out, it's not about language or even credentials," Alex said, turning to face Mark. His eyes held the flicker of realization that had been kindling within him. "It's about growth, isn't it?"

"Definitely. It's like there are these moments that shape us," Mark agreed, nodding slowly.

"Two things, I think," Alex continued, leaning forward, elbows resting on his knees. "Emotional failure or extreme awareness—learning from others. They change a person into something better."

"True," Mark said, pondering over Alex's words. "The roadblocks, the early mornings at the gym, balancing work and study, they've hammered discipline into us."

"Discipline," Alex echoed. "And awareness. Look at what we've learned from Simon, how he runs his business. Or from Emily and Sarah, their drive for engineering. We're not just absorbing knowledge; we're absorbing spirit. Ambition."

"Exactly." Mark's voice was firm, certain. "Our failures hurt but taught us resilience. Our awareness keeps us humble and eager to learn. That's the essence of our journey."

"Too often people forget the power in learning from each other," Alex said, a thoughtful frown creasing his forehead. "They focus inward, but sometimes, looking outward is where you find the answers."

"Or the right questions to ask," Mark added, smiling wryly.

"Right," Alex agreed, a smirk playing on his lips. "Like how to get a girl's number without making a fool of yourself."

"Hey, we survived that too," Mark laughed, the sound rich and warm in the quiet room.

"Survival," Alex repeated softly, the word hanging between them. "That was the beginning. Now we're aiming for thriving."

"Thriving," Mark confirmed, his smile wide. "Together."

They lapsed into silence again, but this time it was comfortable, filled with the unspoken understanding of shared goals and mutual support. Tomorrow would bring another early morning, another day of hard work and discipline, but tonight, they allowed themselves this moment of reflection—a brief pause in the relentless pursuit of their dreams.

Alex leaned back on the worn couch, his gaze drifting to the modest array of potted plants by the window. The quiet hum of the city outside seemed a world away from the contemplative bubble they had created in their small living room.

"Mark," Alex began, breaking the companionable silence, "do you know why I have this huge ambition?"

Mark turned towards him, brow furrowed in curiosity. "No, why?" he asked genuinely intrigued by the sudden shift in Alex's demeanor.

"Because I promised an old friend to get there in 10 years." Alex's voice was barely above a whisper, yet it carried the weight of a vow carved in stone.

"An old friend?" Mark echoed, leaning forward, elbows resting on his knees, recognizing the significance of the revelation.

Alex nodded, his eyes reflecting a mix of nostalgia and determination. "Back home, before I left for Canada. We were kids with big dreams in a small town. He... didn't make it out. But he made me promise that I would chase our dream for both of us."

"Ten years," Mark muttered, the goal suddenly taking on a new gravity. It wasn't just a number anymore; it was a tribute, a deadline woven with loyalty and remembrance.

"Ten years," Alex confirmed, his jaw set firm. "I can't let him down."

"You won't," Mark assured, his tone resolute. "We've got each other's backs, remember? His dream is your dream, and now, it's my dream too. We're in this together, all the way to the top."

"Thanks, Mark," Alex said, a grateful smile touching his lips. "That means everything."

"Anytime, brother," Mark replied, clapping Alex on the shoulder. "Now let's get some rest. Tomorrow, we hit the ground running again."

"Running towards that ten-year mark," Alex added, standing up and stretching.

"Exactly. Towards the future we promised ourselves, and the ones who believed in us," Mark said as they both headed to their respective rooms, their minds already racing ahead to the challenges and triumphs that awaited them on the road to riches.

The morning sun pierced through the blinds, casting a checkerboard of light and shadow across the small living room where Alex sat, knees bouncing with restless energy. Mark paced before him, checking his watch every few seconds as if it could somehow accelerate time. They had been up since dawn, their routine workout at the gym forgone for today's nerve-wracking vigil.

"Did you check your email yet?" Mark asked for the umpteenth time, stopping in his tracks to look over at Alex.

"Every three minutes," Alex replied, barely lifting his gaze from his laptop screen. "Nothing yet."

"Maybe they're just running late with the results," Mark suggested, though his voice betrayed his own anxiety.

"Or maybe they're deciding who gets to deliver the news," Alex half-joked, trying to ease the tension that vibrated between them like a taut string. They shared a brief, tense chuckle before silence reclaimed the room.

"Remember what Simon said?" Mark finally spoke up, referring to their mentor and employer. "'Patience is not simply the ability to wait - it's how we behave while we're waiting.'"

"Simon has a quote for everything," Alex said with a wry smile.

"Because he's seen it all," Mark reminded him. "He started with one Tim Hortons and now he has six. He waited, worked hard—"

"And here we are, following in his footsteps." Alex cut in, his tone more hopeful than he felt. "From two pharmacists turned baristas to... well, whatever comes next."

"Whatever comes next," Mark echoed, nodding firmly. "We'll face it together, rich or not."

"Rich," Alex corrected him, his eyes finally meeting Mark's. "We will be rich. Wealthy in knowledge, experience, and yes, money too. Because we have discipline, remember? That's the most important thing."

"Discipline," Mark repeated, as much to convince himself as to affirm their shared belief.

Their phones buzzed simultaneously, shattering the anticipation that cloaked the room. They exchanged a glance, each finding a reflection of their own apprehension in the other's eyes. This was it—the moment of truth. The culmination of months of relentless studying, working, and planning.

With shaking hands, they reached for their phones. Inhale, exhale. The emails were there, subject lines ominously simple: Examination Results.

"Open it on three?" Alex suggested, his throat tight.

"Three," Mark agreed, and they counted together.

"One. Two. Three."

Fingers tapped screens, and the future unfolded before them in pixels and typography. Their breaths hung suspended, a pair of dreams teetering on the edge of reality.

The silence that followed was deafening, a stark contrast to the cacophony of Toronto's morning rush outside their window. The emails, with their clinical text and heartless delivery, bore the same soul-crushing message: they had failed.

Alex felt as though the ground had been yanked from beneath his feet, a freefall into an abyss he hadn't known existed. Mark simply sat there, his face pale, the light of determination that had always shone in his eyes now dimmed by disbelief.

"Failed," Alex finally whispered, the word tasting like ash on his tongue. "How could we—"

"Stop." Mark's voice was sharp, a blade severing the last threads of hope. "Just stop."

They sat in silence, the magnitude of their disappointment filling the room like a tangible presence, choking and heavy. Plans, dreams, the promise Alex made—everything seemed to crumble around them, leaving behind only fragments of what could have been.

"Mark," Alex tried again, but his friend raised a hand, silencing him.

"Alex, not now. Please." Mark's voice was hollow, the usual warmth replaced with the cold finality of defeat.

Alex respected the plea, sinking back into his chair. The depression settled over them, a thick blanket smothering their aspirations. Neither wanted to talk, to dissect their failure or seek comfort in empty words. They needed to mourn the future they had so meticulously crafted, now just a mirage that dissolved upon contact.

Their shared apartment felt like a mausoleum, housing the ghosts of their past selves—two friends who believed they could conquer a new country, a new life, with nothing but grit and ambition. Now those ghosts wandered aimlessly, haunting the very walls that had witnessed their relentless pursuit of success.

"Maybe tomorrow," Alex thought, but even that sounded like a lie. For the first time since stepping off the plane in Canada, the path ahead was obscured, the ten-year promise broken. What was left for two failed pharmacists in the vast expanse of uncertainty?

"Tomorrow," Mark echoed, as if reading his mind, his gaze fixed on some distant point where hope might still glimmer. But for tonight, they would sit in silence, side by side, lost in the ruins of their dream.

Outside, the city thrummed with life, oblivious to the two friends grappling with their shattered ambitions. The ring of a phone pierced the silence, once, twice, thrice—each call a beacon from a world they were no longer sure they belonged to.

"Shouldn't you answer that?" Alex finally muttered, his voice barely above a whisper, an acknowledgment of the persistence on the other end of the line.

Mark shook his head, eyes never leaving the cold coffee mug he'd been staring into for what felt like hours. "It's them," he said flatly. "Sarah and Emily."

Alex's heart clenched at the mention of Sarah. He had seen his own drive mirrored in her fierce determination, and it had sparked something within him—a shared vision of the future, one where they could both reach their goals side by side. But now, what did he have to offer? A dream deferred?

"They're worried," Alex tried again, reaching toward his own abandoned phone, its screen lighting up with missed calls and unread messages.

"Let them be." Mark's voice was devoid of its usual resolve. "Right now, I can't... We can't..."

The unsaid words hung heavy between them. They couldn't face the pity or the comfort, couldn't pretend that everything was going to be alright when the foundation of their ten-year plan had crumbled beneath them. The discipline, the hard work, the sacrifices—all for naught.

The phones continued their plaintive symphony, a reminder that life was moving forward just beyond their door. Yet here they sat, paralyzed, two statues commemorating a future that would never come to pass.

"Tomorrow," Alex said again, this time a little stronger, as if trying to convince himself. "We'll face it tomorrow."

Mark nodded, and together, they sat in silence, waiting for the sun to set on the longest day of their lives, ignoring the calls that sought to pierce the bubble of their shared solitude. Tomorrow was another day—but tonight, they were alone with their defeat, and that was how it had to be.

The thumping at the door jolted them from their gloomy reverie. Mark and Alex exchanged a look, each silently urging the other to respond, but neither found the strength to rise. The insistent knocking grew louder, more urgent.

"Maybe it's Simon," Alex whispered, a flicker of concern crossing his face. "What if something's happened at work?"

"Simon would call," Mark countered listlessly, though he couldn't help but cast a wary glance toward the entrance.

"Guys! Open up! It's us!" The muffled voices of Sarah and Emily penetrated the thick wooden barrier, laced with worry and determination.

Alex and Mark hesitated—a moment of telepathic debate—before they finally pushed themselves off the couch. They shuffled to the door like shadows drifting through the twilight of their aspirations.

Mark twisted the lock and pulled open the door. The sight of Sarah and Emily, breathless and wide-eyed with concern, was like a gust of fresh air into the stale atmosphere of the apartment. Before either man could muster a greeting or an excuse, they were engulfed in warm, tight hugs.

"Are you guys okay? You didn't answer any calls," Sarah said, pulling back to search Alex's face for answers.

Emily gripped Mark's arm, her eyes scanning his for the truth. "We were worried something had happened."

Their presence, the genuine worry etched into their features, seemed to reignite something within Alex and Mark. Here were two people who cared, who had dashed across the city fearing the worst, not willing to wait another moment for a response. It was humbling and, in some small way, healing.

"We... we got our exam results," Alex admitted, his voice barely above a whisper.

Mark nodded, his gaze dropping to the floor. "We didn't pass."

The silence that followed was filled with unsaid words of encouragement, the shared understanding of disappointment, and the silent promise of support.

"Hey, it happens," Emily finally spoke, squeezing Mark's arm reassuringly. "It doesn't mean it's the end."

Sarah nodded, her hand finding Alex's. "You're both smart and determined. This is just a setback, not a defeat. We'll figure this out together."

In the quiet of the apartment, surrounded by the comfort of friends who refused to let them wallow alone in their despair, Alex and Mark felt the first threads of hope weaving through the fabric of their shattered plans. Tomorrow they would pick up the pieces, but tonight, they were grateful not to be alone.

Sarah's grip tightened around Alex's hand, her resolve as firm as the steel in the city's towering structures they both admired. "You've worked too hard to let this stop you," she said with a conviction that resonated within the walls of the apartment.

"Exactly," Emily chimed in, her optimism infectious. "You guys are not just going to become pharmacists in Canada—you're going to be great ones. One exam doesn't define your future."

Alex met Mark's eyes, and he saw his own disappointment mirrored there. Yet, beneath it, there was something else—a spark reignited by the girls' unwavering belief in them.

"Remember why you started this journey," Sarah continued, her voice soft but strong. "You came here with a dream, and you've been disciplined, hardworking, and dedicated. This is just one step in the journey, and we'll take the next one together."

"Besides," Emily added with a gentle smile, "you've got us now. And we're pretty awesome study partners, if we do say so ourselves."

A small laugh escaped from Mark, the sound brittle but genuine. It was the first hint of lightness in the room since the girls had arrived.

"Alright," Alex said, finding strength in their presence. "We'll try again. We'll study harder, and we won't give up. Not when we have people like you in our corner."

"Damn right," Mark agreed, the corners of his lips tilting upward in a semblance of his usual grin. "Next time, we'll ace it."

The girls exchanged a look, their smiles mirroring the boys'. "That's the spirit," Sarah said. "Now, how about we all get some fresh air? Clear our heads and start planning for round two?"

They all stood, a united front against the temporary defeat. As they walked toward the door, shoulders touching in silent solidarity, the weight of the world felt a little lighter. With each step, the resolve to succeed grew stronger—a testament to the power of friendship and the unyielding determination that had brought them all to this moment.

"Before we hit the books again, I have an idea," Sarah said, pausing by the door and turning to face the somber duo. "Why don't we all go on a camping trip? A bit of time in nature to restore our souls?"

Alex's brows rose slightly, the unexpected suggestion catching him off guard. Mark cocked his head, considering the proposal. The idea of leaving their troubles behind, if only for a weekend, was appealing.

"Nature?" Mark queried, a playful edge returning to his voice. "You mean, actual trees, fresh air, and no textbooks in sight?"

"Exactly," Emily chimed in, her enthusiasm infectious. "A chance to disconnect from all the stress and come back recharged."

"Sounds a bit unconventional," Alex confessed, a small grin tugging at the corner of his mouth. It had been ages since he'd allowed himself the luxury of stepping away from his ambitions, even for a moment.

"Sometimes, the unconventional is exactly what we need," Sarah remarked wisely. "Consider it a strategic retreat. We'll get some perspective, reconnect with ourselves, and then tackle those exams with everything we've got."

Mark nodded slowly, warming up to the idea. "I'm in if you are, Alex." His eyes held a new spark, the wilderness calling to something primal within them both—a yearning for freedom and the simplicity of life beneath the stars.

"Alright," Alex agreed with a deep breath, feeling the weight on his shoulders lift ever so slightly. "Let's do it. Let's go camping."

The girls beamed, already mentally preparing for the trip. As they stepped out into the evening air, the city lights seemed less oppressive, the sky a canvas of possibilities stretching endlessly above them. For the first time in months, Alex and Mark felt like more than just students or aspiring pharmacists— they felt alive, part of something larger and infinitely beautiful.

"Here's to restoring our souls," Mark said, slinging an arm around Alex's shoulder as they followed the girls down the sidewalk, ready to embrace whatever lay ahead.

"Next weekend, then?" Emily confirmed, her voice tinged with excitement.

"Next weekend," Alex and Mark said in unison, their voices firm, resolute. They exchanged glances, a silent pact forming between them. This trip would not be an escape but a chance to refuel their shared dream, to come back stronger. They were warriors in their own right, preparing for the battles ahead.

The city hummed around them, oblivious to the small group's plans, but for Alex and Mark, the promise of the wild was like a beacon cutting through the noise. They could already picture the tranquil lakes, the towering pines, the crackle of a campfire, and the clear night skies.

"Let's make a list of what we'll need," Sarah suggested, ever the planner. "We can divide and conquer the preparations."

"Agreed." Mark pulled out his phone, opening a new note. "Tent, sleeping bags, food supplies, flashlights..."

"Marshmallows," Alex added with a half-smile, momentarily allowing himself a glimpse of normalcy, of carefree moments that had become so rare in their pursuit of success.

"Of course," Emily laughed. "Can't forget those."

They continued to walk, the conversation flowing more easily now, filled with talk of hiking trails and constellations, of disconnecting from the world to reconnect with themselves. And as the city skyline faded behind them, Alex felt a spark of hope ignite within. Maybe this setback was just that—a pause, not an end.

"Next weekend," he repeated softly to himself, the words a mantra of renewal. "We rise again."

As they approached the corner of their street, Mark stopped and turned to face the girls, with Alex standing firmly beside him. The early evening light cast long shadows on the pavement, and a gentle breeze stirred the leaves above them.

"Emily, Sarah," Mark began, his voice firm yet touched by an undeniable warmth, "we just... we can't thank you enough."

Alex nodded, finding strength in Mark's gratitude. "You've been there for us through the grind, the late nights, the stress of it all. And now, when we're at our lowest, you come through with this idea—a way to pull ourselves back together."

"Your support means everything," Alex continued, his eyes reflecting sincerity. "It's easy to get lost in the hustle, to forget that sometimes the best way to move forward is to step back and breathe."

"Absolutely," Mark agreed, glancing at Alex with a shared understanding. They had both been so focused on their ten-year goal that the unexpected failure had hit them hard. But having Emily and Sarah by their sides reminded them that success wasn't just about financial wealth; it was about the richness of relationships, too.

"Next weekend," Emily smiled, her eyes shining with anticipation. "It's a date with nature—and us."

"Can't wait," Sarah chimed in, her enthusiasm infectious.

"Neither can we," Alex replied. "We're really thankful for you girls. We appreciate your help more than you know."

The four of them stood there for a moment longer, basking in the solidarity of their small group. As they continued walking, the air seemed a little easier to breathe, the weight on their shoulders a bit lighter.

"Next weekend," they all echoed, not just as a plan, but as a promise—a promise to rest, to restore, and to return to their dreams with renewed vigor.

Alex's gaze lingered on Sarah, who had been particularly attentive during their time of distress. The quiet concern in her eyes had not gone unnoticed, and as the others chatted about the camping trip logistics, he felt a warmth towards her that went beyond gratitude.

"Hey Sarah," Alex said, his voice low enough to be heard only by her amidst the buzz of conversation. He paused, unsure how to articulate the depth of his appreciation without sounding overly sentimental. "I... I like the way you were there for me—us." His hand gestured vaguely between himself and Mark. "When you hold me, when you show that you're worried... it means a lot."

Sarah's cheeks flushed a soft pink, betraying her otherwise composed exterior. She looked away for a fraction of a second before meeting his eyes again, a mixture of surprise and something gentler in her gaze.

"Alex, I—" she began, but her words trailed off as if she was navigating through her own emotions. "It's just who I am. I care, that's all."

Her response was humble, yet it spoke volumes to Alex. It wasn't just about being physically held; it was the emotional support that came with it—the kind of support that can't be feigned or forced. The kind that was authentic and rare.

"Thank you," he said simply, offering her a smile that communicated more than words could.

Sarah nodded, her embarrassment subsiding under the weight of his genuine thanks. Her eyes danced with unspoken understanding as she replied, "You're welcome, Alex. We're in this together, remember?"

And with that simple affirmation, the seeds of a deeper bond were sown. As the friends continued to plan their respite into nature, the idea of wealth took on a new dimension—one that encompassed the treasures found in human connection and mutual support.

After the heartfelt exchange, the group slowly disbanded, each person peeling away from the collective warmth to face the solitude of their own homes. The city around them seemed to have quieted in sympathy, its usual clamor giving way to a reflective hush.

Mark clapped Alex on the back as they walked down the familiar path that led to their separate apartments. "We'll bounce back from this," Mark said, his voice steady but not without a hint of the struggle they'd been through. "We've got more than just a dream, Alex. We've got people who believe in us."

Alex nodded, feeling the weight of failure being slowly chipped away by the simple acts of kindness and camaraderie they had experienced. "Yeah, we do," he agreed. The depression that had been a suffocating blanket was now receding like a fog at sunrise. It wasn't an instant process; it would take time to fully emerge from the shadows, but the light was undeniably there.

They reached the point where their paths split, and Mark paused, turning to Alex with a resolute look in his eyes. "Tomorrow's another day, brother. Another step towards our goal. We fell, sure. But we get up. We always do."

"Thanks to you, to Sarah, to Emily... to all of us together," Alex added, comforted by the thought that their aspirations were still alive, fueled by shared strength rather than diminished by individual defeat.

"See you bright and early for that run before work?" Mark asked, his eyebrow raised in both challenge and encouragement.

"Wouldn't miss it," Alex replied, the ghost of a smile returning to his face.

With a final nod, they parted ways, each retreating into the sanctity of their own thoughts. As Alex closed his apartment door behind him, he felt a sense of calm settle over him. He realized that while wealth was still the destination, the journey had become richer with every stumble and each supportive hand offered along the way.

In the quiet of his room, Alex allowed himself to envision the future—not just the material success, but the personal growth and the bonds formed. Yes, they had failed an exam, but they hadn't failed each other. That realization alone was enough to stoke the dying embers of ambition within him.

"Ten years," he whispered to himself, a silent vow echoing against the walls. "The climb continues."

And with that thought, Alex laid down, allowing sleep to claim him, confident that when dawn broke, he and Mark would rise once more, ready to face whatever challenges awaited them—richer already in ways that mattered most.

The morning of the camping trip dawned crisp and clear, a welcome reprieve from the emotional turbulence of the past weeks. Alex was already up, packing his duffel bag with the essentials: a sleeping bag, a portable stove, and a first aid kit, ingrained habits from a life dedicated to both preparedness and healthcare.

"Think we'll need this much food?" Mark's voice rang out from the kitchen, where he stood surveying the cache of supplies they'd amassed for the weekend. Protein bars, bags of trail mix, and pre-packed meals were laid out on the counter like rations for an army.

"Better to have too much than too little," Alex responded, zipping his bag shut. "Especially since we're relying on our own cooking skills this time."

"Speak for yourself," Mark chuckled, tossing a bag of marshmallows into a cooler. "I've been mastering the art of campfire cuisine via online tutorials."

"Let's hope those tutorials included how to start a fire without burning down the forest," Alex teased, hoisting his duffel over his shoulder and joining Mark in the kitchen.

The girls' car, a sturdy SUV fit for the rugged landscapes north of Toronto, honked outside, signaling Sarah and Emily's arrival. The two friends exchanged a look, their spirits buoyed by the thought of escape into nature's embrace—a chance to reset and rejuvenate.

"Alright, let's do this," Mark said, grabbing his own gear and heading for the door. Alex followed suit, taking one last glance at the apartment before stepping out into the new day.

The air had that fresh bite that hinted at the approach of spring, invigorating and full of promise. As they loaded their equipment into the back of the car, Alex couldn't help but feel grateful—not just for the opportunity to get away, but for the company he was with. Sarah and Emily were quickly becoming more than just gym acquaintances; they were allies in the quest for balance and happiness.

"Everything set?" Emily asked from the driver's seat, her smile as warm as the sun climbing higher in the sky.

"Ready as we'll ever be," Alex confirmed, closing the trunk with a satisfying thud.

"Then let's hit the road," Sarah added, the anticipation clear in her voice.

The journey north was filled with laughter and stories, the landscape outside the windows shifting from urban sprawl to verdant forests and rolling hills. Alex felt the tension of the city's pace dissipate with each mile, replaced by a sense of freedom and possibility.

As they drove, Mark pulled out the piece of paper with their 12-month plan scribbled on it—now slightly crumpled and frayed at the edges. He glanced at Alex, a silent agreement passing between them. They would revise it together later, perhaps by the campfire, under a blanket of stars. For now, it was enough to know the paper held dreams not yet deterred by setbacks.

"Here's to reaching new heights," Mark said, lifting an imaginary glass in toast.

"And to the people who climb with us," Alex added, feeling a camaraderie that went beyond words.

Their destination was now only a few winding roads away. A weekend of reflection and recovery awaited them, nestled in the heart of the Canadian wilderness. As they continued their drive, guided by the unwavering compass of friendship and ambition, Alex knew that true richness lay in moments like these—shared, savored, and utterly priceless.

The car finally turned off the main road onto a gravel path, the tires crunching over stones as they wound their way deeper into the wilderness. The dense canopy of trees above them filtered the sunlight into a mosaic of dancing patterns on the forest floor. Alex rolled down the window, letting in the crisp, pine-scented air that filled his lungs with each breath. He felt alive, more connected to the present moment than he had been in months.

"Almost there, guys!" Emily called from the driver's seat, her tone buoyant.

Mark nodded, folding the plan and tucking it away safely in his backpack. He caught Alex's eye and grinned. "No books, no counters, no prescriptions for two whole days," he said. Their shared experience at the pharmacy had become a routine they both knew needed a break from.

"Yep," Alex agreed, "just us and nature." He appreciated the irony that despite their ambitions, they were finding solace in simplicity. Perhaps this was the universe's reminder that wealth wasn't solely about financial gain, but also about rich experiences and relationships.

As the car came to a stop at the edge of a serene lake, Mark and Alex eagerly hopped out. They stretched their limbs, stiff from the drive, and surveyed their temporary home. The water was a mirror reflecting the sky, and the surrounding trees stood like sentinels guarding a sacred place.

"Time to set up camp," Mark announced, reaching for the tent bag. They worked together seamlessly, the tent rising quickly under their practiced hands. The physical activity was a welcome change from the mental exertions of studying and planning.

With the campsite established, they sat on the edge of the dock, their feet dangling over the cool water. They shared easy conversation, interspersed with comfortable silences. Laughter echoed across the lake as Sarah and Emily joined them, the four friends basking in the collective sense of relief from life's pressures.

"Who's ready for some fun?" Alex asked, a mischievous glint in his eyes. In response, Mark launched into an exaggerated tale of their most memorable gym mishaps, sending them all into fits of laughter.

As the sun began its descent, casting golden hues across the landscape, they prepared for an evening by the fire. There was something primal about the flickering flames that spoke to Alex's soul, reminding him that the journey to wealth was not just about the destination but also about the paths taken and the memories made along the way.

"Tomorrow, we hike to the lookout point," Sarah suggested, and they all agreed enthusiastically.

"Tonight, we make the best s'mores ever," Emily declared, brandishing marshmallows like a culinary challenge.

"Challenge accepted," Alex replied, feeling a lightness in his spirit. For now, plans and ambitions could wait. This weekend was about living fully in the moment, about being rich in joy and companionship. And as the stars emerged one by one, like beacons of hope in the darkening sky, Alex knew they had achieved just that.

The first light of dawn filtered through the canvas of their tents as Alex stirred from his slumber. The air was heavy with the scent of pine and earth, a natural perfume that invigorated the soul. He unzipped the tent and stepped out into the cool morning, finding Mark already up, stretching his limbs with a series of practiced movements.

"Morning," Alex greeted, his voice still hoarse with sleep.

"Ready to conquer the day?" Mark replied, cracking a smile as he gestured towards the lake, where a thin mist hovered above the water's surface.

"Absolutely," Alex said, his energy building with each breath of fresh air.

They began an impromptu game of tag, darting between trees and leaping over exposed roots, the childhood joy of play reigniting within them. Sarah and Emily emerged from their own tent, laughter spilling from them like sunlight as they joined in the frolic.

Before long, they were all breathless, cheeks flushed with exertion and happiness. They collapsed onto the grass in a tangle of limbs, the sky above a canvas of soft blues and pinks as the sun climbed higher.

"Best way to start the day," Emily said, her eyes sparkling with mirth.

"Agreed," Alex responded, feeling his heart swell with gratitude for this simple moment of bliss.

"Let's not forget the hike though," Sarah reminded them, ever the planner.

"Give us five minutes to catch our breath," Mark bargained, rolling onto his side to face the girls.

"Five minutes," Sarah conceded with a mock stern look, which quickly melted into a warm smile.

Lying there amidst the sounds of nature and the easy camaraderie, Alex realized that richness wasn't just about wealth in the traditional sense—it was also about these moments of pure, unadulterated joy. As they eventually rose to prepare breakfast before their hike, he knew that no matter what the future held, the memories forged here would be a treasure more valuable than any currency.

After a hearty breakfast that tasted better in the crisp outdoor air, they shouldered their backpacks and set off on the hiking trail that curled around the campsite like an inviting serpent. The forest welcomed them with the symphony of rustling leaves and birdsong, the ground a mosaic of earthy colors.

Alex led the way, his strides confident but respectful of the natural world they traversed. Mark was beside him, map in hand, occasionally glancing at it before looking up to take in the scenery. Sarah and Emily followed close behind, pointing out various flora and fauna, sharing snippets of information about each species.

"Did you know that pine trees can live to be over a thousand years old?" Emily mused aloud, her gaze lingering on a particularly grand specimen.

"Imagine the stories it could tell," Alex replied, lost in thought. He felt a deep connection to the land underfoot, a reminder of the steady passage of time and the fleeting nature of human endeavor.

As they climbed higher, the terrain grew more challenging. Roots became natural steps, rocks obstacles to navigate. Every so often, they would stop to rest, drinking in the views that stretched out before them: rolling hills, distant lakes shimmering like jewels, and the vast expanse of wilderness that made their everyday worries seem insignificant.

"Look at us, city folks getting our hands dirty," Mark joked, wiping his brow. He had always been the one to find humor even when faced with adversity, and Alex appreciated that about him now more than ever.

"Feels good, doesn't it?" Sarah said, her cheeks rosy from the climb. She caught Alex's eye, and he nodded in agreement, feeling a kinship with her adventurous spirit.

The hike wasn't just a physical journey; it was a metaphor for their shared ambitions. Each step was progress, each obstacle a challenge to overcome—much like their dreams of riches not just in wealth, but in experiences and achievements.

As the day wore on and the sun began its descent, they found a clearing with a view that stole their breath away. They settled there, each lost in their thoughts, and as the sky turned to fire with the setting sun, Alex realized that this was wealth. This moment, this bond, this unspoken promise to support each other through thick and thin—that was the true treasure they were all seeking.

The twilight crept in, a gentle reminder that the day's adventures were drawing to a close. As the first stars emerged, Alex and Mark gathered wood together, moving with a silent, practiced teamwork born from years of shared goals and mutual support.

Sarah and Emily brought over kindling, their laughter and conversation weaving through the air like music. The fire pit, a shallow grave dug earlier, awaited its purpose. With a few strikes of flint on steel, sparks leaped onto the tinder, catching hold and breathing life into a small but growing flame.

"Here we are," Alex said, his voice soft yet carrying in the hush of the surrounding woods. He placed another log onto the fire, watching the flames lick eagerly at the fresh fuel. "We've come a long way since landing in Toronto."

Mark nodded, poking at the fire with a stick, encouraging it higher. "From two pharmacists dreaming of wealth to... well, still dreaming, but with better company." His smile was wry, but his eyes held a spark akin to the embers before them.

"Sometimes," Emily interjected, handing out marshmallows on sticks, "wealth isn't measured by your bank account, but by moments like these."

They all fell into a comfortable silence then, each lost in the dance of flames that cast warm glows upon their faces. The fire crackled, a cozy soundtrack to their collective introspection. In its light, they saw not merely the flicker of shadows, but the reflection of their journey—the discipline, the hardships, the unwavering determination to succeed—and how those experiences had melded them closer.

"Tomorrow's another day," Sarah murmured, leaning back to gaze up at the stars. "Another chance to chase our dreams."

"That's right," Alex agreed, feeling a resurgence of that familiar ambition. "And we'll be ready for it, no matter what comes our way."

Together, they sat around the fire, bound by more than the shared warmth; they were united by a vision of the future, one where success was defined not just by their careers or bank balances, but by the richness of life's journey and the people who walked it with them.

The night deepened, the stars above becoming ever more vivid as the fire's glow settled into a soothing lull. A gentle breeze whispered through the trees, carrying with it the serenity of the wilderness. In this moment, stripped of the city's clamor and the relentless pursuit of their ambitions, Alex and Mark found a peace they hadn't realized they'd been missing.

"Look at that constellation," said Sarah softly, pointing towards the heavens where a cluster of stars seemed to sketch out an intricate pattern against the night sky. Her voice, tinged with wonder, drew Alex's gaze upwards. He moved closer to Sarah, her presence a comforting weight beside him.

"Ursa Major," he identified, tracing the outline with his finger in the air.

"Very good," she smiled, leaning into his side. Her arm wrapped around his waist, a gesture of affection that sent a warm flush through him. Alex returned the embrace, feeling a connection that went beyond words, beyond the dreams of wealth and success. It was as if Sarah's hug bridged the gap between the life he had envisioned and the one unfolding before him—one filled with unexpected tenderness.

On the other side of the fire, Emily nudged Mark playfully. "You know, for two guys fixated on conquering the world, you're pretty good at this whole relaxation thing."

Mark chuckled, the sound mingling with the crackle of the burning wood. "Well, we've got excellent teachers." He turned to Emily, his eyes reflecting the dance of the flames. She scooted closer, her head coming to rest on his shoulder. Mark's arm instinctively curled around her, pulling her in for a hug that felt like a promise—a silent vow to remain steadfast not just in ambition but in nurturing the bonds they had formed under the canopy of stars.

As the night wore on, the foursome shared stories and laughter, each tale weaving them tighter into the fabric of friendship and romance. The fire eventually dwindled, its embers glowing softly like distant galaxies, but the warmth between them remained undiminished.

"Life's full of surprises, isn't it?" Alex mused aloud, more to himself than anyone else.

"Yep," agreed Mark, his gaze lingering on Emily's face, illuminated by the dying light. "And I wouldn't have it any other way."

In the heart of nature, surrounded by the tranquility of the woods and the company of those who mattered, Alex and Mark understood that richness wasn't a destination but a journey—a path walked with the right people, under the right stars. And as they sat there, enveloped by the night's embrace, they realized that perhaps they were richer than they had ever imagined.

The tranquility of the forest was a soothing balm to their bruised ambitions. As dawn's first light pierced the veil of darkness, Alex stirred from his restful slumber. Beside him, Sarah lay serene, her breaths deep and even. Across the dying embers of the fire, Mark and Emily were huddled in a similar cocoon of contentment. The night had been an unexpected reprieve, a gentle reminder that life still held moments of pure, unburdened joy.

Alex sat up, stretching his arms towards the awakening sky, the cool morning air invigorating his senses. Mark followed suit, rubbing sleep from his eyes. They exchanged a look, one that carried a shared resolve to face the coming challenges head-on, but not before cherishing the precious respite they had found here, in this temporary wilderness retreat.

"Morning already?" Mark yawned, a smile tugging at his lips.

"Looks like it," Alex replied, his voice low, not wanting to disturb the peaceful slumber of the girls.

Together, they commenced the routine of breaking camp with practiced efficiency, folding tents and rolling sleeping bags with the sort of silent communication born of deep friendship. The campfire was cold now, its ashes scattered and buried with respect for the natural haven that had sheltered them.

Sarah and Emily awoke to the sounds of clinking camping gear and whispered strategy for the journey back to the urban jungle of Toronto. They emerged from their tent, eyes bright and spirits lifted by the previous night's connection. The four friends shared a simple breakfast, each bite infused with the flavor of the great outdoors and the sweet aftertaste of newfound affection.

"Back to reality, huh?" Emily said, tying her hair into a ponytail, readying herself for the return trip.

"Reality isn't so bad when you've got the right people to share it with," Alex responded, his smile genuine, as he looked around at the group.

"Let's pack up and hit the road," Mark announced, clapping his hands together with decisive energy.

They worked as a team, loading backpacks and dousing the last traces of their campsite. The girls' car, parked a short hike away, awaited them like a chariot ready to whisk them back to the concrete embrace of Toronto.

"Thanks for this," Sarah said, her hand brushing against Alex's as they walked. "I think we all needed it."

"More than you know," Alex agreed, the gratitude in his heart reflecting in his eyes.

By the time they reached the car, the sun was fully aloft, casting a golden glow over the landscape. The drive back was quiet, contemplative, each lost in thought but bound together by the shared experience of the weekend.

Toronto's skyline eventually crept into view, a stark contrast to the idyllic setting they were leaving behind. Yet, as they drove into the busy city, there was no sense of loss, only anticipation for what lay ahead. With renewed vigor and the support of one another, Alex and Mark were ready to tackle their dreams once again, knowing that true wealth lay not just in the riches they sought, but in the relationships they nurtured along the way.

The steady hum of the car engine mixed with the distant sounds of the city as it came to life, the routine cacophony of urban existence enveloping them like an old familiar song. Alex caught Sarah's reflection in the side mirror, her face alight with a soft smile that seemed to hold the secrets of serenity.

"Let's do this camping thing like every month or two," Sarah suggested, breaking the silence. "It's like a reset button for the soul, you know?"

Mark nodded in agreement from the driver's seat. "A chance to breathe away from the grind. I'm in."

"Me too," Emily chimed in from beside him, her voice tinged with the same excitement that had carried them all weekend.

Alex smiled, his thoughts aligning with theirs. "Yeah, it's like we can leave everything behind, even if just for a little while. It keeps us grounded."

"Exactly," Sarah said, turning to lock eyes with Alex. "We can refresh ourselves, keep our dreams alive without burning out. Balance is key."

"Balance," Alex repeated, the word resonating within him. They had all experienced the highs and lows of chasing ambition, but it was moments like these that truly enriched the journey.

"Here's to making memories and recharging spirits," Mark declared, lifting an imaginary glass as they approached the outskirts of the city.

"Cheers to that," they all echoed, laughter spilling into the car, a shared commitment to not only their individual goals but to the collective adventure that lay ahead.

The city skyline came into view, a familiar sight that usually signaled the return to routine, but this time it felt different. The concrete jungle didn't seem as daunting after spending the weekend surrounded by nature's grandeur.

"Home sweet home," Mark murmured as he navigated the streets with a practiced ease.

"Thanks for driving, Mark," Emily said, her hand finding his on the console.

"Anytime," he replied, giving her hand a gentle squeeze.

Alex glanced out the window, watching as the urban landscape whisked by. The trip had indeed been a balm to their bruised spirits, a much-needed interlude from the relentless pace of their lives. The failure of their exams had hit them hard, but now there was a renewed sense of hope, an inner strength rekindled by the support of Sarah and Emily.

"Thank you both," Alex said sincerely as they pulled up to their apartment building. "This weekend was exactly what we needed."

Sarah met his gaze, her eyes reflecting understanding and warmth. "We all needed it," she admitted. "It's not just about picking each other up when we fall. It's about sharing these moments, growing together."

"Couldn't have said it better myself," Emily added, as they unloaded the gear from the trunk.

"Let's get everything inside and then grab some dinner," Mark suggested. "My treat."

"Sounds like a plan," Alex agreed.

As they ascended the steps to their apartment, a comfortable silence enveloped the group—a silence that spoke volumes about the bond they shared. They were four individuals united by aspiration and affection, a small tribe within the vastness of Toronto.

"Here's to new souls and great trips," Alex said, holding the door open for the others.

"Here's to us," Sarah replied, stepping past him with a smile that promised more adventures to come.

"Here's to life," Emily added, her voice echoing in the stairwell.

The door closed behind them with a soft click, sealing away the world for a moment longer as they reveled in the camaraderie and the promise of tomorrow.

"Remember that squirrel?" Mark chuckled as they began unpacking their camping gear in the living room, the laughter coming easy now. "I've never seen a creature with such a death wish for granola."

Alex grinned at the memory, the image of the audacious little rodent trying to make off with their breakfast etching a permanent place in his mind. "Yeah, and Sarah's impression was spot-on," he added, placing the rolled-up tent back in its bag.

"Hey, I do a pretty mean squirrel," Sarah protested playfully, striking a pose that had them all laughing again.

"Emily's fire-making skills though," Mark said, gesturing appreciatively at Emily. "We would've had a very different night without your pyrotechnic prowess."

"Teamwork makes the dream work," Emily replied, winking.

The atmosphere was light, the energy in the room almost palpable as they cleaned up. Alex felt it—an invigorating rush of vitality coursing through him, the weight of their past failures lifting, if only for the moment.

"Guys," Alex said once the last of the equipment was stowed away, "this trip didn't just give us a break. It gave us a reminder." He looked around at his friends, their faces expectant. "We set out with dreams in our hearts, and we've been knocked down hard. But we're here, we're still standing, and we're not alone."

"Absolutely," Mark agreed, nodding emphatically. "We came here to make something of ourselves, to build a future. And that's exactly what we're going to do."

"Back to the grind tomorrow," Alex said, determination solidifying his resolve. "Back to studying, to working, and yes, to dreaming. We have goals to reach, and this"—he gestured to encompass the room, the memories, the shared experiences—"is just part of our journey."

"Couldn't have put it better myself," Mark said, clapping Alex on the shoulder. "Let's get some food and then rest up. We've got a big day ahead."

They left the apartment in high spirits, the camaraderie between them an unspoken vow to support each other through thick and thin. The city lights twinkled like distant stars as they walked to their favorite diner, each step a reaffirmation of their commitment to their dreams.

"Here's to chasing riches of all kinds," Mark said as they settled into a booth at the diner.

"Rich in experience, rich in friendship, and yeah, rich in the bank too," Alex added, raising an imaginary glass.

"To us," they all said in unison, and to anyone watching, it was clear: these four were more than friends. They were a force to be reckoned with, united by ambition and bound by love.

Alex and Mark ambled back to their apartment in comfortable silence, the cool night air whispering around them like a promise. The streets of Toronto were quieter now, the hustle of the day giving way to the calm of the evening. Streetlights cast elongated shadows as they walked, their forms merging and separating with each step.

The key turned in the lock with a familiar click, and they entered the sanctuary of their shared space. It was a modest apartment, but it represented so much more than just four walls and a roof; it was the starting block from which they would launch themselves towards their dreams.

"Home sweet home," Mark murmured appreciatively, kicking off his shoes by the door.

"Yep," Alex agreed, following suit. He stretched out his arms, rolling his shoulders to release the tension of the day. "Can't believe how much energy those girls have—camping two day, then hitting the books again the next."

"Or that they're as crazy about camping as we are about our ten-year plan," Mark chuckled, flopping onto the sofa. He picked up a notepad from the coffee table—their plans and aspirations scrawled across its pages—and flipped through it thoughtfully.

"Speaking of which," Alex said, sitting down beside him. "We should review our steps tomorrow, make sure we're on track."

"Absolutely," Mark agreed, nodding. "But tonight, we rest. We've earned it."

They prepared for bed in a routine that had become second nature, a quiet efficiency in their movements. The bathroom light flicked off, and the apartment settled into darkness save for the faint glow of street lamps filtering through the curtains.

In the stillness, Alex found himself reflecting on the day's events—the laughter, the warmth, the shared understanding with their new friends. It was a welcome respite from the relentless pursuit of their ambitions, a reminder that life wasn't just about the destination, but also about appreciating the journey.

"Goodnight, Mark," Alex whispered across the room, where the soft sound of steady breathing told him his friend was already drifting off to sleep.

"Night, Alex," came the drowsy reply.

And with that, they surrendered to slumber, the challenges and triumphs of tomorrow waiting patiently for their return. In the world of dreams, they were already rich men—not just in wealth, but in spirit, friendship, and resolve. Tomorrow, they would wake ready to face the world once more, their bond unbreakable, their determination unwavering. Tonight, they rested, the architects of their own destiny.

The shrill alarm pierced the silence of dawn, and Alex's hand shot out from under the covers to silence it. His eyes blinked open to the dim light of early morning filtering through the blinds. Beside him, Mark groaned, a muffled protest against the intrusion of daybreak.

"Time to rise, my friend," Alex said with a hint of encouragement as he swung his legs over the edge of the bed.

Mark responded with a grunt but pushed himself into a sitting position, rubbing the sleep from his eyes. They moved in tandem, a practiced routine that had become their daily ritual: dress, hydrate, and gather their gym gear.

Today was no different from any other, despite the disappointment they had recently faced. Their drive to succeed had not waned; if anything, their resolve had deepened. The sting of failure had been soothed by support and camaraderie, and now it fueled them.

At the gym, weights clanked and machines whirred as Alex and Mark fell into the rhythm of their workout. Each lift, each step on the treadmill, was a metaphor for their journey—pushing against resistance, enduring when every fiber begged for respite. Sweat beaded on Alex's forehead, the burn in his muscles a familiar comfort.

"Remember, discipline is key," Mark panted between sets, echoing their shared mantra.

"Discipline and protein," Alex shot back with a smile, recalling their commitment to a diet that complemented their training.

Their laughter echoed in the gym, a sound of resilience. After their session, they showered, changed, and headed to work at Tim Hortons, greeting Simon with a nod as they clocked in for their shift. The familiar scent of coffee and baked goods enveloped them, another layer of their new life in Canada.

There was little time for idle chatter as they navigated the morning rush, but in quieter moments, they exchanged knowing glances—a silent conversation about the future they were building together.

The workday gave way to evening, and then it was time to hit the books. Their study space was a fortress of concentration, textbooks and notes spread around them like ramparts. They quizzed each other, challenged each other, striving for mastery over the material that stood between them and their pharmacist licenses.

"Remember why we're doing this," Alex said as they wrapped up a particularly grueling study session.

"To build our empire," Mark replied without missing a beat.

"Exactly," Alex confirmed. "We'll pass this exam, get our degrees recognized, and then the real work begins."

They packed away their study materials, a sense of accomplishment mingling with exhaustion. But beneath the fatigue, there was a pulse of excitement—tomorrow was another opportunity to move closer to their goal.

"Let's do this," Mark said, determination etched in his features.

"Let's make our dream a reality," Alex agreed, feeling the weight of their ambitions as a mantle, not a burden.

As they settled into bed that night, the quiet hush of their apartment was a stark contrast to the vibrant energy that thrummed within them. They closed their eyes, minds already racing toward the sunrise that would herald a new day of possibilities.

"Goodnight, Mark."

"Goodnight, Alex."

Sleep came easily, the restorative balm for warriors in the midst of battle, dreams their temporary refuge until they would wake to fight once more.

The dawn crept in with a subtle brightness that filled the room, casting a warm glow on the two friends who had already begun to stir from their rest. Alex blinked open his eyes, adjusting to the light, and turned to see Mark already sitting up, rubbing the sleep from his face.

"Morning," Alex mumbled, his voice heavy with sleep.

"Morning," Mark replied, a slight grin forming as he stretched out his stiff muscles.

They rose from their beds, bodies still weary but minds alert, knowing well the routine that awaited them. A quick breakfast, a brisk jog to the gym—these were the constants upon which they built their foundation for success.

But today felt different. Today, there was an air of reflection, a momentary pause in their relentless pursuit. They finished their workout in silence, each man lost in thought. The clanking of weights and the rhythm of treadmills around them faded into a background hum, secondary to the internal dialogues they each conducted.

After showering and dressing, they found themselves standing in their apartment, the day's schedule yawning wide before them. It was then that Alex turned to Mark, a look of resolve mingling with fatigue etched across his features.

"Mark," he began, his voice steady despite the uncertainty that quivered at its edges, "let's have a rest for a week, then we start studying again."

Mark considered Alex's words, the suggestion of a respite both tempting and terrifying. They had been pushing relentlessly, fueled by ambition and the fear of failure. Yet, the allure of a brief hiatus, a chance to recharge and regroup, held a promise of renewed vigor.

"Are you sure?" Mark asked, the weight of their shared goal pressing down upon him. "We can't afford to lose momentum."

Alex nodded, conviction solidifying within him. "I am. We've been going non-stop, and if we burn out now, all our efforts will be for nothing. We need this, Mark—a short break to clear our heads and come back stronger."

Mark searched Alex's eyes, looking for any sign of doubt or hesitation, but found none. Instead, he saw the same unyielding determination that mirrored his own—the drive that had propelled them from their homeland to Canada, from pharmacists to aspiring entrepreneurs.

"Alright," Mark conceded, the hint of a smile creeping onto his lips. "One week. But then it's back to the grind, no excuses."

"Agreed," Alex said, the pact between them sealed.

For a moment, they allowed themselves the luxury of imagining a week without textbooks, without the relentless ticking of the clock. In that brief interlude, they were not students or future businessmen; they were simply two friends, navigating the complexities of life in a foreign land, leaning on each other for strength.

"Let's make the most of it," Mark suggested, his spirit visibly lifted by the prospect of rest.

"Definitely," Alex replied, a sense of relief washing over him. "We'll come back fresh and hit the books harder than ever."

With their decision made, they stepped out of their apartment, the city of Toronto sprawling before them—a canvas on which they would paint their dreams, bold and unfading. For now, though, they would take a breath, embrace the present, and ready themselves for the challenges that lay ahead.

The week of reprieve passed like a fleeting dream, a temporary escape from the relentless pursuit of their ambitions. Alex and Mark had allowed themselves to breathe, to live without the omnipresent weight of textbooks and medical journals. They laughed more freely, slept without the haunting specter of exams, and for a moment, life was simple.

But as the new dawn crept through the blinds of their shared apartment, casting a grid of light across the room, the undeniable truth settled back upon their shoulders: it was time. Time to rekindle the flame of discipline that had brought them this far, time to chase down the future they had envisioned for themselves.

Sitting at their modest kitchen table, which doubled as their study desk, Alex cracked open the heavy cover of a pharmaceutical text, its pages dense with knowledge yet to be conquered. The scent of fresh coffee permeated the room, a familiar comfort and an unspoken signal that the hiatus was over.

"Today's the day, Mark," Alex said, his voice steady, instilled with a quiet confidence. "We start again, but this time, we're going all the way."

Mark nodded, his eyes focused on the array of notes and books before him. He pulled out a pen, the click echoing in the stillness of the morning—a clarion call to action. "We've got this, Alex. We're not just preparing for an exam; we're building our future, one study session at a time."

They fell into a rhythm, the turning of pages and scribbling of notes creating a symphony of progress. As the sun climbed higher, bathing the room in golden warmth, a silent covenant was forged between them. They would not falter, not now, not ever. Every word absorbed, every concept mastered, brought them closer to the wealth and success they yearned for—a testament to their unwavering ambition.

Alex glanced across the table at Mark, catching the intense concentration etched on his friend's face. He felt a surge of camaraderie, knowing they shared more than a goal; they shared a journey—one marked by sacrifice, resilience, and an unbreakable bond.

"We'll do it next time," Alex reaffirmed, more to himself than to Mark. "We'll pass, we'll thrive, and we'll look back on today as the moment we turned the tide."

"Absolutely," Mark agreed, without lifting his gaze from the intricate diagrams before him. "We've learned, we've grown, and there's no stopping us now."

Together, they delved deeper into the world of medicine, their dreams fueling a tireless pursuit of excellence. In the quiet of their apartment, with only each other and their aspirations for company, Alex and Mark began anew, their ambition unwavering—a beacon guiding them toward the riches of knowledge and the promise of a prosperous future.

Alex's voice broke through the stillness once again, solidifying their resolve. "Hey, Mark," he said, his tone imbued with a steely determination that left no room for doubt. "We will not have a rest until we pass the qualifying exams."

Mark raised his head, meeting Alex's eyes squarely. In that look, there was a mutual understanding that transcended words—an unspoken pact that they would push through exhaustion, frustration, and any obstacle that stood in their way.

"Rest can wait," Mark replied firmly. "Our future doesn't."

With that, they returned to their studies, their focus sharpening like a blade honed for battle. The pages of their textbooks were well-thumbed, the margins filled with annotations and highlights—a map of their intellectual journey. They parsed through complex pharmaceutical information, challenged each other with questions, and debated points until concepts became clear as crystal.

As evening crept in and the shadows grew long across the floor, neither man showed signs of fatigue. They had each other, and that was more than enough to keep the fires of motivation burning bright.

Hours passed, and the city outside their window transitioned from the bustle of daylight to the hushed tones of night. Still, Alex and Mark remained at their table, surrounded by papers and books, their spirits undimmed. Their dreams of wealth and success were not mere castles in the sky; they were foundations built on hard work and unwavering discipline.

And so, they continued, chapter by chapter, problem by problem, forging ahead with the knowledge that every effort brought them one step closer to their ten-year goal. In the silent camaraderie of shared ambition, they found strength, and in the relentless pursuit of their dreams, they found purpose.

The days melded into weeks, and the weeks into months. The cycle of waking, studying, working, and training became their life's rhythm, a symphony that played to the tune of their unwavering resolve. Their apartment, once an empty canvas of two hopeful immigrants, was now a war room where strategies for success were plotted with meticulous care.

Alex's eyes would occasionally drift to a photograph pinned above his desk—a reminder of his old friend and the promise he had made. It spurred him on, adding fuel to his already burning desire to succeed. He knew Mark shared a similar drive, each feeding off the other's determination in an unspoken pact of brotherhood.

The relentless winter gave way to a gentle spring, and with it came the day they had both been preparing for—exam day. As they stepped out of their building into the crisp morning air, there was a palpable tension between them, a mix of nerves and excitement.

"Today, we conquer," Mark said with a quiet intensity as they joined the stream of commuters.

"Or we learn to conquer another day," Alex replied, equally resolute. They knew the path to riches was not linear, but they were ready to face whatever result came their way.

As they traveled towards the exam center, submerged in the city's pulse, they shared a silent vow. This was more than just passing an exam; it was about proving to themselves that their dreams were valid, that their sacrifices mattered, and that their ambition was not in vain.

Arriving at the testing venue, they were greeted by the hum of anxious candidates, each absorbed in last-minute revisions and whispered prayers. Alex and Mark exchanged a look of solidarity before joining the throng, their steps echoing on the polished floors.

They found their designated seats in the examination hall, a sea of desks neatly arranged in solemn rows. The proctor's voice cut through the murmurs, signaling the start of the test.

Pens poised, Alex and Mark flipped open the first page of the exam booklet. Years of study, months of sacrifice, all led to this moment. They began to write, their hands steady, their minds clear. They were ready.

Hours passed in a blur of concentration. Graphs, formulas, and case studies filled page after page as Alex and Mark worked through the questions with methodical precision. They had prepared for this, revisiting every topic until they knew it by heart. The exam was tough, but so were they.

As the final minutes ticked away, they reviewed their answers, ensuring no careless mistake could rob them of their hard-earned victory. Their focus was unwavering, a testament to the discipline that had become their creed.

"Time," the proctor finally called out, snapping the room back into the present. Pens dropped, and a collective sigh of relief swept through the hall. Alex closed his booklet, feeling a weight lift off his shoulders. Beside him, Mark did the same, stretching his arms with a satisfied grin.

They filed out with the other test-takers, the tension dissipating into excited chatter. In the lobby, Alex clapped Mark on the back, sharing an exhilarated smile.

"We did it," Alex said, his voice brimming with pride.

"We did," Mark agreed, his eyes gleaming with certainty. "No matter what the results are, we walked out of there knowing we gave it everything."

Their confidence wasn't just bravado; it was rooted in months of relentless study, the support of each other and their friends, and the unwavering belief in their ten-year plan. They had faced the challenge head-on and emerged smiling, comfortable in the knowledge that they had performed to the best of their abilities.

Alex and Mark stepped out into the bright afternoon sun, the city's heartbeat syncing with their own. Today, they felt invincible, their dreams within touching distance. Tomorrow, they would continue their journey, but today, they basked in the glow of a battle well fought, certain in their hearts that success was on the horizon.

"Let's call the girls," Mark suggested, his voice tinged with excitement. "They've been part of this journey too."

"Absolutely," Alex agreed as they walked down the sidewalk, their strides purposeful yet relaxed.

Mark pulled out his phone and dialed Emily's number, holding the device to his ear. The dial tone hummed a brief prelude before her voice came through, clear and expectant.

"Hey, Emily," Mark greeted, unable to keep the triumph from his voice. "We just finished our exam, and... I'm sure this time we'll pass. It's not like before."

On the other end, Emily's response crackled with enthusiasm. "I knew you guys could do it! Sarah and I never doubted for a second."

"Thanks, Em," Mark said, the corners of his mouth lifting into a smile. "Hearing that means everything."

Alex watched as Mark's eyes softened, the connection between him and Emily palpable even through the digital divide. It was more than just sharing news; it was confirmation of their shared resilience, a testament to the bond that had formed among them.

"Let's meet up later and celebrate?" Mark suggested, hope coloring his voice.

"Count us in!" came Emily's reply, the sound of her laughter like music to their ears.

"Great," Mark replied, his heart lighter, the future brighter. "We'll see you then."

As they hung up, the two friends exchanged a look of mutual understanding. They had navigated the trials together, bolstered by companionship and the pursuit of a common dream. Now, with renewed vigor and hearts full of hope, they were ready to face whatever came next, knowing that no matter the outcome, they had each other—and that made all the difference.

Alex clapped Mark on the back, the motion brimming with silent camaraderie. "Let's get out of this place," he said, eager to leave the exam hall that had been their battleground for the past hours.

They spent the afternoon in a heady mix of relief and anticipation. The city around them seemed to hum with the same vibrancy that coursed within their veins. They walked streets lined with promise, explored shops as if seeing them for the first time, and laughed at jokes that weren't particularly funny but hilarious to them in their current state of joy.

By the time they met up with Sarah and Emily, the sun was dipping low, painting the sky a palette of oranges and purples. The girls were waiting outside a small café, their faces lit by the golden hour glow.

"Hey, champions!" Sarah greeted, her voice a melody of excitement.

"Hey yourself," Alex replied, unable to suppress a smile as he caught Sarah's eye. There was something in her gaze, an echo of the pride he felt.

Mark and Emily shared a brief, electric embrace, the kind that spoke volumes without a word being uttered.

"First round of coffees on us," Emily declared, ushering them into the café with an arm sweep that was both grand and playful.

The café was cozy, a little haven away from the world where the scent of roasted beans was strong and comforting. They chose a table by the window, bathed in the remnants of daylight, and settled into a comfortable rhythm of conversation and laughter.

"Here's to hard work and second chances," Mark toasted, lifting his mug.

"To resilience," added Sarah, her eyes twinkling.

"And to friendship," Alex concluded, feeling the weight of the moment, the sense of unity among them.

They clinked their cups, the sound crisp and clear, a symphony of hope and determination. It was easy to forget everything else when surrounded by people who understood the depth of your struggle and the height of your aspirations.

After the café, they decided to keep the evening light and carefree. They played arcade games at a nearby entertainment center, battled it out over air hockey, and raced against each other in virtual car chases. Each victory was celebrated with high-fives and each loss with good-natured ribbing. The spirit of competition was alive but friendly, a reflection of their journey together.

As the night drew to a close, they found themselves strolling along the waterfront, the city lights reflecting off the water like scattered jewels. Conversation turned to dreams and plans, to what the future might hold, but always with the underlying knowledge that they would face it together.

"Today was perfect," Emily murmured, leaning her head on Mark's shoulder.

"Perfect indeed," Alex agreed, his gaze lingering on Sarah, who smiled back softly.

They knew there would be challenges ahead, but for now, they reveled in the simple joy of one day spent with no worries, just fun—a much-needed respite before they returned to the pursuit of their dreams.

The dawn light trickled into the sparsely furnished apartment, casting a soft glow on the two figures stirring from their slumber. The digital clock on the nightstand read 5:00 AM, its persistent beep cutting through the silence like a starting pistol for the day ahead.

Alex groaned, his eyelids heavy with the remnants of sleep but his mind already tuning to the frequency of ambition. He watched as Mark, ever the early riser between them, stretched and shook off the warmth of the bed.

"Hey Alex," Mark said, tying his sneakers with swift, practiced motions. "You know what we have to learn about trading and investing? If we do that with our degree, that will be perfect. But let's learn them after we start working as pharmacists."

Alex sat up, the gears in his head beginning to turn. "Yeah, diversifying our knowledge is key.

It's not just about earning but making what we earn work for us." His voice was thick with sleep but underscored by an alert sharpness that came from years of dreaming alongside Mark.

"Exactly," Mark replied, standing up and heading towards the kitchenette to grab their pre-workout shakes. "We can't rely solely on one source of income if we want to reach our goals."

Their shared apartment, though modest, was a fortress of their aspirations. The walls were lined with schedules and study materials, charts tracking their progress, and a whiteboard filled with motivational quotes. The two friends moved in sync, a routine perfected by months of repetition—gym, work, study, repeat.

They dressed in silence, each lost in thoughts of financial strategies and investment portfolios. The dream of wealth wasn't just about luxury; it was about security, freedom, and the ability to make a difference. They both knew that expanding their expertise beyond pharmacy was another rung on the ladder they were determined to climb.

"Let's crush this workout," Mark said as he tossed Alex his shake, the clinking of the bottles a familiar rallying cry.

"Then it's back to the grind," Alex replied, downing the protein-rich liquid in a few large gulps. He could almost taste the future they were fighting for, and it was sweeter than any shake.

With their gym bags slung over their shoulders, they locked the door behind them, stepping out into the still-quiet streets of Toronto. As they made their way to the subway station, the city around them slowly awakened, mirroring their own rise from obscurity to success—a journey they were more determined than ever to complete.

The shift at Tim Hortons passed in a blur of steaming coffee and the clatter of cups. Alex and Mark served customers with mechanical efficiency, their minds already on the pages awaiting them, the formulas and drug interactions they'd need to master for the exam. When Simon, their boss, popped in to check on things, he gave them an approving nod. He had become more than just an employer; he was a mentor, an unwitting part of their grand plan.

"Good work today, guys," Simon said, his voice carrying over the hum of the restaurant. "Keep this up, and you'll run the place soon."

Alex exchanged a glance with Mark, a silent acknowledgment of their shared ambition. They didn't intend to run a Tim Hortons; they aimed much higher. But every step counted, every shift was another coin in their jar of dreams.

"Thanks, Simon," Mark responded. "We're doing our best."

"Off to study again?" Simon asked, already knowing the answer.

"Every day gets us closer," Alex replied with a determined smile.

As the clock struck four, Alex and Mark hung up their aprons and said their goodbyes. They stepped out into the afternoon sun, fatigue tugging at their muscles but not their spirits. They felt the weight of the textbooks in their backpacks, a reassuring presence that spoke of progress and persistence.

"Ready to dive back in?" Alex asked, squinting against the light as they made their way to the library.

"Always," Mark answered. "We've got no time to waste."

At their usual table, surrounded by stacks of reference materials, the two friends settled into the familiar silence of study. They flipped through pages, scribbled notes, and quizzed each other on pharmacological principles. It was a dance of intellect, each step taking them closer to their goal.

Hours ticked by, marked only by the occasional stretch or coffee break. The world outside faded away, leaving only their shared vision and the relentless pursuit of knowledge. Their focus was unwavering, their dedication unmatched. This exam was more than a hurdle; it was the gateway to everything they had planned.

"Remember, discipline is the bridge between goals and accomplishment," Mark muttered, quoting one of the mantras from their whiteboard.

"Exactly," Alex agreed, his fingers flying over his calculator. "We're building that bridge, one study session at a time."

As the library's closing announcement echoed through the room, Alex and Mark gathered their materials. They were mentally exhausted but fulfilled. Each night like this was a step toward wealth, toward the life they had envisioned when they first stepped foot in Canada.

"Same time tomorrow?" Mark asked as they exited the library.

"Without fail," Alex confirmed, his resolve as solid as the ground beneath their feet.

They split with a fist bump, two friends united by a dream that was slowly but surely becoming reality. The road ahead was long, but they had each other—and that was all the motivation they needed.

Sunlight filtered through the curtains, casting a warm glow across Alex's face as he lay sprawled on his bed, the tranquility of sleep still clinging to him. His phone buzzed insistently on the nightstand, a sharp contrast to the peaceful morning. Groaning, he reached for it, his eyes squinting against the sudden flood of light from the screen.

"Mark," he mumbled, thumbing the speaker button. "This better be good."

"Check your email, Alex!" Mark's voice crackled with excitement, a stark departure from their usual pre-coffee grumblings.

With a quizzical frown, Alex dragged himself up and shuffled over to his laptop. The familiar blue glow welcomed him as he logged in, his heart rate inching higher with every passing second.

"Okay, I'm in," Alex said. "What am I looking for?"

"Your future, man! The results!"

His inbox was a mosaic of spam and newsletters, but one subject line stood out, bold and unopened: Exam Results Notification. He clicked it, holding his breath.

"Come on, come on," he muttered under his breath, the loading symbol mocking him with its slow spin.

Then, there it was—the email that held their fate.

"Dear Candidate, we are pleased to inform you..."

Alex didn't need to read any further. A whoop of joy erupted from him, loud enough to echo through the quiet apartment. He was on his feet now, adrenaline coursing through his veins.

"Mark, we did it! We passed!"

The cheer that came through the phone was triumphant, the sound of ten years' worth of dreams starting to crystallize into reality. It was the sound of discipline paying off, of early mornings at the gym and late nights at the library converging into this single, victorious moment.

"Did you ever doubt us?" Mark's laugh was infectious, and Alex found himself laughing too, the sound bright and hopeful.

"Never," Alex replied, his mind already racing ahead to the next steps, to trading and investing, to opening their own pharmacy. But for now, this victory was enough—a promise that their ambition was not misplaced, that their hard work had not been in vain.

"Let's celebrate tonight," Mark said, the smile evident in his voice. "We've earned it."

"Agreed," Alex responded, his gaze drifting to the window where the city bustled below, oblivious to the monumental shift that had just occurred in apartment. Toronto was their playground now, and they were ready to conquer it, together.

"Let's take the girls out," Alex suggested, already picturing Sarah's smile when she heard the news. "They've been with us every step of this journey."

"Exactly what I was thinking," Mark replied. "I'll call Emily and let her know. Meet you at our usual spot in an hour?"

"Perfect. See you then." Alex hung up, his heart still racing. He took a moment to let it all sink in—the countless hours spent memorizing drug interactions, the mechanisms of action, the side effects—all leading to this.

He glanced around the small apartment he shared with Mark, the tidy space a testament to their discipline. Textbooks lay stacked on the coffee table, highlighted and annotated, while gym bags were neatly tucked away, ready for the next early morning workout. Everything had its place, including their dreams.

With renewed energy, Alex pulled on his best shirt, the one reserved for special occasions. He studied himself in the mirror, noting the healthy glow of his skin, a byproduct of their nutritious diet and exercise regimen. The reflection that stared back at him was that of a man who knew where he was going, of someone who would not—could not—be stopped.

He met Mark outside, and together they walked to the quaint cafe where they'd first bonded with Sarah and Emily over coffee and dreams. The winter air was brisk, invigorating, as if it too was celebrating their success.

Their laughter filled the evening as they recounted tales from their exam preparations, the late nights and early mornings, the nervousness that had gripped them just before entering the examination hall. It felt like a lifetime ago now, even though only hours had passed since they received the results.

Sarah and Emily arrived, faces bright with anticipation. The girls had become so much more than just partners in study sessions; they were confidantes, supporters, integral pieces of their lives in Canada.

"Tell us already!" Emily urged, her eyes sparkling with excitement.

"We passed!" Mark announced, unable to keep the pride from his voice.

The shrieks of delight from Sarah and Emily melded with the ambient sounds of clinking glasses and soft music. They celebrated with a toast, their glasses raised high, the sweet clink echoing like a bell of triumph.

"Here's to dreams coming true," Alex said, his eyes meeting Sarah's across the table. "To never giving up, and to the best is yet to come."

The night unfolded with an ease that only comes with deep-seated contentment. They dined, laughed, and shared stories, basking in the collective joy of overcoming hurdles together. When the meal concluded, they strolled through the streets, the city lights casting an ethereal glow on their path.

"Every month or two, we should do something like this," Sarah suggested, her hand finding Alex's as they walked. "To remind ourselves of how far we've come, and how far we still have to go."

"Agreed," Alex said, squeezing her hand gently. "Celebrations like this are our milestones. They mark the journey, not just the destination."

As the night drew to a close, they parted ways with promises of future gatherings and adventures. Alex and Mark returned to their apartment, the day's emotions ebbing into a peaceful, satisfied exhaustion.

"Tomorrow, we start the next chapter," Mark said, his voice steady with resolve.

"Tomorrow," Alex agreed, already half-asleep, his mind drifting off with visions of pharmacies bearing their names, of wealth not just in finances but in friendships and fulfillment. Tomorrow, they would return to their disciplined routine, but tonight, they rested as victors. Tonight, they were rich in every way that mattered.

The first light of dawn crept through the blinds, casting a soft glow across the room where Alex and Mark lay sprawled in their respective beds. The celebrations of the previous night still lingered in the quiet air, 3a silent testament to their recent triumph. But as the clock ticked on, the real world beckoned, demanding their attention with the unforgiving persistence of reality.

Alex's alarm chirped insistently, rousing him from a contented slumber. He reached out, silencing it with a practiced tap before rubbing the sleep from his eyes. There was a moment, just a heartbeat, where he allowed himself to savor the sweet victory of the night before. But it passed quickly as he swung his legs out of bed and planted his feet firmly on the ground.

"Time to get back to it," he muttered to himself, the words a familiar mantra.

Mark, already stirring, echoed the sentiment with a grunt of agreement as he too rose to face the day. The two friends shared a look of mutual understanding; there was no need for grand speeches or motivational talks. They knew the path they had chosen was one of relentless pursuit, and the routine was their compass.

In the kitchen, they moved with efficiency, fueling their bodies with protein-rich breakfasts and strong coffee. Notebooks lay open on the table, a tangle of medical terms and diagrams scrawled across the pages, waiting to be conquered once more. Their conversation was sparse, focused, each phrase sharpened by determination.

"Pharmacokinetics today," Alex announced, tapping a page filled with complex equations.

"Right." Mark nodded, taking a last sip of his coffee before standing up. "Let's not forget to review those new drug interactions, too."

They cleared the table swiftly, their movements synchronized by months of shared routines. It wasn't just about passing exams or earning degrees anymore – it was about forging a future with their own hands, piece by piece.

As they settled into their study session, the world outside hummed with life, but within the walls of their apartment, time seemed to slow down. The only sounds were the rustle of pages turning and the occasional murmur of recited facts.

Focused, they delved deeper into their studies, each fact memorized, each concept understood, building the foundation of their dreams with unwavering discipline. This was the reality of their ambition: not glamorous, not always thrilling, but essential. It was the grind that would elevate them, the diligence that would eventually see their vision come to pass.

"Remember," Mark said during a brief pause, glancing over at Alex, "it's the daily steps that lead to giant leaps."

Alex simply nodded, a small smile playing on his lips. They were in this together, side by side, both anchoring and propelling each other forward. The dream of wealth was still ten years away, but with every page turned and every formula learned, they were inching closer to the summit of their aspirations.

And so, surrounded by textbooks and ambition, Alex and Mark got back to work, their spirits undeterred, their will unbroken. The road to riches was long, but they had taken the first steps. Now, there was no looking back. Only forward, toward the future they were determined to build.

The sun had dipped below the horizon when the knock at their door disrupted the silence. Alex and Mark exchanged a look, both puzzled by the unexpected intrusion. They weren't due to meet anyone at this hour, certainly not Simon, who typically communicated through calls or texts.

"Who could it be?" Alex whispered as he stood up, stretching his limbs, stiff from hours of sitting.

"Maybe the girls forgot something last time they were here?" Mark suggested with equal curiosity.

Alex approached the door and opened it to reveal Simon, the owner of the Tim Hortons where they worked. His presence was unexpected, but not unwelcome; they owed much of their current stability in Canada to him.

"Simon," Alex greeted, ushering him inside. "This is a surprise. What brings you here at this hour?"

"Boys," Simon began, his tone amiable yet carrying an undertone of seriousness. "I've been thinking. You guys are pharmacists, and while I appreciate your hard work at my restaurants, it's clear you're overqualified for pouring coffee."

Mark joined them, wiping his hands on a towel. "We do what we have to," he said, a firm nod underlining his words. "But we're studying to get our degrees recognized here. It's just a matter of time."

"Which is why I'm here," Simon said, leaning against the back of their worn-out couch. "I have a friend who runs a pharmacy nearby. They're looking for assistants—pharmacy assistants. It's closer to your field, and it might even help with your exams."

Alex and Mark glanced at each other, the gears turning in their heads. The opportunity was unexpected, a stroke of luck that seemed too good to pass up.

"Wouldn't that require our Canadian certifications?" Alex asked cautiously, not wanting to get his hopes up only for them to be dashed by red tape.

"No, not as assistants," Simon clarified. "You'd be working under a licensed pharmacist, but it would give you relevant experience here. And," he added with a knowing smile, "it pays better than flipping doughnuts."

"It sounds like just what we need," Mark admitted, a spark of hope igniting in his eyes. "Practical experience and better pay could accelerate our plans."

"Exactly," Simon agreed. "I thought it might help with your ten-year goal."

"Thank you, Simon," Alex said sincerely. "This means a lot to us. We'll definitely look into it. Right, Mark?"

"Absolutely," Mark concurred, his earlier fatigue forgotten in light of this new possibility. "It's a step up, a chance to get closer to our dream."

"Great," Simon said, satisfied. "I'll put in a word for you two. Expect a call soon."

With handshakes and grateful smiles, they saw Simon out, closing the door behind his departing figure. The room felt different now, charged with potential.

"Looks like discipline is paying off sooner than expected," Alex remarked, a glint of excitement in his eye.

"Let's make the most of it," Mark replied. "For ourselves, for our future."

And with renewed vigor, they turned back to their books. Tomorrow held the promise of new opportunities, and they were ready to embrace them.

The next morning, just as the first tendrils of dawn crept through the blinds, Alex's phone rang. He was already awake, the anticipation of Simon's promise stirring him from sleep hours earlier. Rubbing the sleep from his eyes, he glanced at the caller ID—a number he didn't recognize—and answered with a cautious, "Hello?"

"Is this Alexander?" The voice on the other end was tinged with age, its timbre carrying the weight of years and wisdom.

"Yes, speaking," Alex replied, sitting up straighter.

"This is Magie, owner of the Pharmacy. Simon spoke highly of you and your friend Mark. I understand you're both pharmacists looking for an opportunity to work in a pharmacy setting here in Canada?"

"That's correct, Ms. Magie," Alex said, a surge of excitement making his heart race.

"Please, call me Magie. I'm looking for two dedicated individuals to assist in my pharmacy. It's a small team, but we pride ourselves on providing personal care to each customer that walks through our doors."

"We would be honored to join your team, Magie," Alex affirmed, feeling Mark's eager gaze upon him from the adjacent bed.

"Good," she replied with a tone that suggested a smile. "Can you start next week? We'll need to go over some formalities, of course, but I trust if Simon vouches for you, it's more than enough for me."

"Absolutely, we can start whenever you need us," Alex assured her, exchanging a triumphant look with Mark.

"Perfect. Come by the pharmacy tomorrow afternoon, and we'll discuss everything in person. I look forward to meeting you both."

"Thank you so much. We'll see you then." Alex ended the call, his pulse thrumming with anticipation.

"Was that her?" Mark asked, barely containing his own excitement.

Alex nodded, a broad grin spreading across his face. "We've got the job, Mark. We're going to be pharmacy assistants!"

Mark let out a whoop of joy, leaping from his bed. They exchanged a high-five, the sound echoing in the quiet apartment like a harbinger of the success they were determined to achieve.

"Discipline, my friend," Mark said, his eyes alight with determination. "It's starting to pay off."

"Let's not forget persistence and ambition," Alex added, his mind already racing ahead to their new beginning. "Together, they're the perfect prescription for success."

In that moment, standing in their modest living room, the future seemed brighter than ever. With discipline as their guide and ambition as their drive, Alex and Mark were ready to take on the next chapter of their journey to prosperity.

The next day dawned crisp and clear, a typical Toronto morning with the city slowly rousing to life. Alex and Mark set out early, the excitement of their impending meeting with Magie infusing an energetic spring in their step. They walked side by side, their breaths visible in the cool air, discussing strategies and reviewing their plans for the future.

"Remember, we must be candid about our situation," Alex reminded Mark as they neared the pharmacy. "We are committed to becoming licensed pharmacists here, and that's a non-negotiable part of our agreement."

"Agreed," Mark nodded. "We need this job, but not at the cost of our main goal. Magie needs to understand that."

They arrived outside the quaint pharmacy nestled in a busy strip of local businesses and paused, taking a moment to appreciate how far they had come and through the large storefront windows, they could see rows of neatly arranged products.

"Ready?" Alex asked, his hand on the door handle.

"Ready," Mark confirmed, and together they stepped inside.

The bell above the door chimed cheerfully as they entered. The interior was warm and inviting, with a faint medicinal scent that brought a sense of familiarity and comfort. An elderly lady looked up from behind the counter, her eyes sharp and assessing behind thin-rimmed glasses.

"Alex and Mark, I presume?" she said, a trace of a smile tugging at the edges of her lips.

"Yes, ma'am," Alex replied. "You must be Magie."

"That I am," she affirmed, walking around the counter to greet them. Her handshake was firm, belying her age. "Simon speaks very highly of both of you. Now, tell me about your plans for licensure."

As they explained their dedication to studying for the Canadian pharmacy board exams, Magie listened intently, nodding along. It was evident that she appreciated their ambition and the clarity of their plan.

"Your determination is commendable," Magie said once they finished. "I've been looking for assistants who have more than just technical skills. Your drive to succeed will serve you well here."

"Thank you," Mark said. "We're eager to learn from you and contribute to the pharmacy in any way we can."

"Good," Magie replied. "We'll start with training you on our systems and protocols. And I'll do my part to support your studies. After all, one day, you might be running a place like this yourselves."

Her words cemented their resolve, reinforcing the vision that had brought them to Canada. As they discussed work schedules and responsibilities, Alex felt gratitude surge within him—gratitude for Simon's referral, for Magie's trust, and for the friendship beside him that had made all of this possible.

"Let's get started, shall we?" Magie proposed, her energy seemingly boundless. "There's no time like the present to build toward the future."

And with that, Alex and Mark followed her into the heart of the pharmacy, ready to absorb every lesson, every experience that would bring them closer to their dream. Their journey had taken a significant step forward, and though the road ahead was long, they faced it united, with steadfast discipline and irrepressible ambition.

The training session was exhaustive, covering the ins and outs of pharmaceutical operations. They touched on inventory management, prescription processing, customer service protocols, and even the nuances of insurance claims. Alex and Mark felt their brains swell with information, but they relished the challenge.

"Pay close attention to the dosage instructions," Magie said, guiding them through a mock consultation. "It's not just about dispensing medicine; it's about ensuring the well-being of those who trust us with their health."

Alex nodded, scribbling notes as Magie spoke. He glanced at Mark, who was equally engrossed in the learning process. It was a silent agreement between them that no detail was too small, no task too menial. They were building a foundation, one brick at a time.

As the day waned, shadows grew long across the pharmacy floor, and the stream of customers slowed to a trickle. Magie finally called an end to the session.

"Alright, gentlemen, I think that's enough for today," she declared, a soft smile on her face. "You've both done exceptionally well. Keep this up, and you'll be ready in no time."

"Thank you, Magie," Alex replied, his voice weary but spirited. "We appreciate this opportunity more than you know."

"Indeed," Mark added, stretching his arms above his head. "We won't let you down."

"See you bright and early tomorrow morning," Magie said as she walked them to the door.

Stepping outside, the cool evening air was a balm to their overworked minds. They walked side by side in comfortable silence, each lost in thought about the future. The city lights twinkled like distant stars, illuminating paths to countless destinations. For Alex and Mark, their destination was clear, but the path was theirs to forge.

"Two weeks of training," Mark murmured as they reached the subway station. "Then the real work begins."

"Two weeks to learn everything we can," Alex agreed. "And then we apply it, every day, until we're where we want to be."

"Discipline is our ladder to success," Mark said, a determined glint in his eye.

"Exactly," Alex said, smiling despite the fatigue. "Discipline, and maybe a little bit of dreaming too."

They descended into the station, ready to rest and recharge. Tomorrow promised another demanding day of training, but they welcomed it. With each new piece of knowledge, with each skill mastered, they were inching closer to their goal. Their dream of wealth wasn't just about money; it was about the richness of purpose, the wealth of self-made success.

Home was a modest apartment, a far cry from the luxurious life they envisioned. But as they closed the door behind them, leaving the world outside, they felt a deep sense of peace. Here they could relax, if only for a few hours, before rising again to meet the demands of their relentless ambition.

Alex's fingers hovered over his phone, the light from the screen casting a soft glow in the dim room. He tapped the contact name 'Sarah' and waited as the call connected, the rings punctuating the silence of their apartment.

"Hey, Alex," came Sarah's warm voice, a balm to the fatigue that clung to his bones.

"Hey," he replied, a smile curving his lips. "I just wanted to tell you about today. The training was intense, but informative. We're learning so much."

"Tell me everything," Sarah urged, her enthusiasm infectious.

He recounted the day's events, describing how he and Mark absorbed every detail, every instruction given by their trainers. She listened intently, her occasional hums of encouragement a reminder of her unwavering support.

"Sounds like you're on the right track," she said once he finished. "I'm proud of you, Alex. Both of you."

"Thanks, Sarah. It means a lot," he said, the gratitude evident in his voice. "Having your support, it's... well, it's everything."

There was a moment of silence, the kind filled with unspoken words and shared understandings.

"Alex," Sarah breathed out, her voice suddenly serious. "There's something I need to say. I've been feeling this for a while now, and I think you should know—I love you."

The words hung in the air, carrying a weight that seemed to shift the very atmosphere. He felt a swell of emotion, a mix of surprise and profound happiness. This confession was an unexpected gift, a treasure he hadn't known he was seeking.

"Sarah," he whispered, his own heart racing with the truth of his feelings. "I love you too."

On the other end of the line, he could almost hear her smile, the warmth in her tone wrapping around him like a comforting embrace. In that moment, despite the exhaustion, despite the long road ahead, Alex felt an immense sense of contentment. Her love was another beacon in his journey, a shining reminder that no dream was pursued alone.

They talked into the night, their conversation meandering from dreams to mundane daily occurrences—a comfortable rhythm established between two hearts beating in sync. Eventually, as the moon carved its arc across the starlit sky, fatigue wrapped its gentle arms around Alex. They bid each other goodnight, a promise of tomorrow lingering in their farewell.

"Sleep well, Sarah," he murmured, the line already silent, her presence felt like an echo in the room.

"Goodnight, Alex," she had said, her voice a soothing lullaby that guided him into slumber.

The next day dawned bright and clear, painting Toronto with strokes of warm gold and crisp azure. It was one of those mornings that held the subtle promise of endless possibilities. Alex stretched his limbs, feeling the pleasant ache of yesterday's training—a physical reminder of progress.

"Morning," Mark grumbled from his bed across the room, rubbing the sleep from his eyes.

"Morning," Alex replied, already reaching for his phone to check the time. They had a routine to stick to—a discipline that was non-negotiable.

As they prepared breakfast, the scent of toast mingling with the aroma of fresh coffee, Alex recounted the conversation he had with Sarah. He spoke of her belief in them, her encouragement, and finally, her declaration of love.

"Sarah's amazing, man," Alex said, a soft smile on his face. "She said she loves me."

Mark paused, his mug halfway to his lips. "Wow, that's... that's huge, Alex."

"Yeah, it is." Alex's smile grew wider. "And you know what? It's just more motivation. Her belief in me... in us... it's like she's become a part of this dream. The reason behind my goal isn't just for me anymore. It's for us—for our future."

Mark nodded, understanding written all over his face. "Having someone like that in your corner—it changes things. Makes the tough days easier to get through."

"Exactly," Alex agreed, his determination solidifying. "We're going to make it, Mark. For ourselves, for our partners, for the lives we want to build."

They clinked their mugs together, a silent toast to goals set and the shared journey ahead. With the support of people like Sarah and Emily, their resolve took on a new depth, fortified by love and the shared vision of success.

"Alright," Mark said after a moment, setting down his empty mug. "Let's hit the gym, then tackle the day. We've got work to do, my friend."

"Let's do it," Alex replied, ready to face the challenges ahead with renewed vigor.

The crisp morning air bit at their cheeks as Mark and Alex made their way to the gym, each step a testament to the discipline they had forged over months of early rises. The city was just beginning to wake, the sky painted in hues of pink and orange that heralded the new day.

"Sarah's really something," Mark broke the silence, his breath visible in the cool air. "And Emily... she's been incredible too."

Alex glanced over, catching the hint of vulnerability in his friend's tone. "You've got it bad for her, huh?"

Mark let out a chuckle, shaking his head with a rueful grin. "Yeah, I guess I do. She's strong, independent, driven... reminds me a lot of us when we first started out on this journey."

"Seems like you two are a good match then," Alex nudged him playfully with his elbow.

"Maybe." Mark's gaze drifted towards the horizon, where the sun was now peeking above the skyline. "But I've made a decision. I'm going to tell her how I feel about her—after I pass the second exam."

"Is that so?" Alex raised an eyebrow, impressed by the resolve in his friend's voice.

"Yep," Mark affirmed. "It's all about priorities, right? Our dream comes first. Once I've got that piece of paper confirming I'm a licensed pharmacist here, then I'll have the space to focus on... well, on other important things in life."

"Sounds like a plan," Alex nodded in approval. "One thing at a time, one goal after another."

"Exactly," Mark agreed, his steps gaining momentum as they approached the gym. "We can't lose sight of what we came here for. But knowing there's more to look forward to— that's not a distraction. It's fuel."

"Fuel for the fire," Alex echoed, feeling the truth of those words resonate within him.

They entered the gym, greeted by the familiar clank and whir of machines and weights. Here was where they honed not only their bodies but also their minds, preparing themselves for the rigors of the exams and the demands of their future businesses. Every rep, every set, was a stepping stone toward their shared vision of success.

As they began their workout, the determination that had brought them to this country, that had seen them through job searches and intense study sessions, coursed through their muscles. And now, love intertwined with ambition, adding a new layer of complexity and reward to the already intricate tapestry of their aspirations.

"Let's crush this workout," Mark said, his voice steady and sure.

"Then it's back to the grind," Alex added, equally resolute.

"Ten years," Mark reminded him, a fire in his eyes that matched the rising sun.

"Ten years," Alex agreed. And in their hearts, they knew they were building something far richer than wealth—they were building lives full of purpose, passion, and love.

Exiting the gym, the brisk Toronto air felt invigorating against their heated skin. The city's pulse was a rhythm set by ambition and relentless motion—a symphony they were determined to join as more than mere background instruments.

"Remember," Mark said as they walked toward the subway station, "it's not just about passing exams. It's about building the life we promised ourselves."

Alex nodded, feeling the weight of his backpack heavy with textbooks. "We've come too far to be sidetracked by one night of fun."

"Exactly," Mark affirmed. They descended into the belly of the subway, the fluorescent lights stark against the evening's encroaching darkness.

The train arrived with a whoosh, doors sliding open to welcome them. As they settled into their seats, Alex's phone vibrated in his pocket. The screen lit up with Sarah's name. He hesitated for a moment before answering.

"Hey, Sarah," he greeted, his voice steady despite the flutter in his stomach.

"Alex! Emily and I are going to this amazing party tonight. You guys should come!" Sarah's excitement bubbled through the phone.

He glanced at Mark, whose expression echoed his own resolve. "I wish we could, but we can't tonight. We have a lot of studying to do."

There was a pause, then Sarah's understanding sigh. "You two are so driven. Alright, rain check then?"

"Rain check," Alex confirmed, feeling a twinge of regret even as he knew their choice was the right one.

"Good luck with the studying. Call me tomorrow?"

"Will do," Alex replied, ending the call with a small smile. Beside him, Mark was scrolling through digital flashcards, already a step ahead.

As the train rumbled on, the world outside blurred into streaks of light and shadow. Inside, two friends sat side by side, their focus unwavering, their dreams undimmed. The promise of wealth and success lay on the horizon, but only if they refused to be pulled away by the sirens' call of instant gratification.

"Back to it, then," Mark said, breaking the comfortable silence.

"Back to it," Alex agreed, opening his book to the next chapter.

The train sped on into the night, carrying them closer to their ten-year goal, while the city above continued its dance, oblivious to the quiet dedication unfolding in its depths.

Months of relentless hard work and fervent studying had passed since that disciplined decision to skip the party. The day they had been inching towards with painstaking precision finally dawned, a culmination of all their sacrifices—the exam day.

Alex woke up before the alarm, his heart thrumming with a cocktail of nerves and excitement. He turned to see Mark already up, practicing deep breathing exercises to calm his racing mind.

"Today's the day, man," Alex said, his voice steady despite the butterflies in his stomach.

"Let's crush it," Mark replied, with a conviction that seemed to electrify the air around them.

They followed their morning routine like clockwork, each step feeling surreal, as if they were walking through a familiar dream. Breakfast was consumed in companionable silence; each bite loaded with the weight of the momentous day ahead.

At the examination center, they joined a sea of eager faces, but there was an unspoken confidence between them. They had not only prepared for the test, they had lived and breathed the material, letting it seep into the marrow of their existence.

"Remember, it's just another day at the gym," Mark whispered as they entered the hall, a reference to their countless early mornings spent building both mental and physical strength.

"Another set of weights," Alex agreed with a nod, grateful for the analogy that grounded him.

The questions on the exam were challenging, designed to weed out those less determined, less disciplined. But Alex and Mark tackled each one with a surgeon's precision, their pencils dancing across the answer sheets, translating months of study into decisive marks of ink.

As the final seconds ticked away, they exchanged a look, no words needed. They laid down their pencils simultaneously, a silent symphony of synchronization that had become second nature.

Walking out of the exam center, they allowed themselves a moment of relief. The sun seemed to shine brighter, and the world appeared sharper, as if they were seeing everything for the first time.

"We did it," Alex said, his smile a mirror of Mark's.

"Onto the next challenge," Mark replied, slinging an arm around Alex's shoulder. The path ahead was clear, their steps light with the buoyancy of certainty. They had faced the test not just with hope, but with the assurance of two men who knew that their dreams were not hinged on mere chance, but on the foundation of unwavering effort and discipline.

"Tonight, we celebrate this victory," Alex declared. "Tomorrow, we conquer the next."

"Absolutely," Mark agreed, the energy of accomplishment radiating from him. "We've earned that much."

They stepped out into the bustling Toronto streets, the city's rhythm matching the pulse of their own hearts. They walked with purpose, their strides long and confident. They had come to this land as newcomers, but now they strode through it as conquerors of their own fate.

"Remember when we were memorizing drug interactions and dosage calculations?" Alex mused, a chuckle escaping his lips. "It felt like climbing a mountain."

"Mountains are there to be climbed," Mark said, his eyes alight with the reflection of their shared ambition. "And look at us now, standing on the summit, ready for the next peak."

The cool breeze carried with it the scents of the city—the distant aroma of coffee, the urban tang of metal and concrete—and beneath it all, the faintest hint of possibility. It was the scent of new beginnings, of doors opening.

"Let's not forget what got us here," Alex reminded them both, his voice taking on a solemn note amidst their triumph. "Discipline. Without it, none of this would have been possible."

Mark nodded, his expression earnest. "Discipline is the bedrock. And our dreams, well, they're the blueprint."

As they continued their walk, their conversation turned to plans for the evening— nothing extravagant, just a simple celebration.

A quiet acknowledgment of the milestone they had reached together. They knew the journey was far from over, but for tonight, they could bask in the glow of a job well done.

"Tomorrow, we'll wake up early, hit the gym, and keep moving forward," Alex said, the future calling to him with open arms.

"Exactly," Mark concurred, his thoughts already turning to the steps ahead. "We'll pass, I can feel it. And then we'll take everything we've learned and build something lasting. For ourselves, for those we care about."

They arrived at their apartment building, the familiar sight welcoming them home. Tonight, they would rest, their minds and bodies at ease, secure in the knowledge that they had given their all.

"Next time we walk out of an exam room," Alex said, his hand on the door, preparing to enter their shared sanctuary, "it'll be as licensed pharmacists. And that's just the beginning."

"Absolutely," Mark echoed, "the very beginning of everything we've ever wanted."

As the door closed behind them, the two friends stepped into their home, their bond unspoken but as tangible as the walls around them. They had each other, their shared dreams, and a tenacious grip on the future that awaited them.

With the evening air crisp and filled with the electric buzz of Toronto nightlife, Alex and Mark strolled down the vibrant streets lined with glowing signs and lively chatter. Their strides were buoyant, fueled by the adrenaline of completion and anticipation for what was to come.

"Let's give Sarah and Emily a call," suggested Alex, his thumb hovering over the screen of his phone. "It's time we let loose a little."

"Definitely," agreed Mark, his eyes sparkling in the neon lights. "They've been there through it all, they should be part of this celebration."

The phone rang briefly before a voice answered, cheerful and expectant. Alex's face broke into a wide grin as he relayed the day's triumphs, the excitement palpable in his voice. The girls' elation came through clearly, their words quick and eager.

"We aced it, or at least it feels like we did," Alex exclaimed, the pride in his achievement ringing clear. "We can't wait to see you guys. How about we meet up ? Celebrate properly?"

"Sounds perfect!" came the enthused reply from the other end. The promise of a night spent among friends, reveling in the hard-earned pause from their relentless pursuit of success, was irresistible.

"Great, we'll see you there in an hour," said Mark, already picturing the cozy interior of their favorite bar, where many a plan had been hatched over chilled pints and warm laughter.

The bar welcomed them with its familiar convivial ambiance, a mix of soft lighting and the murmur of patrons enjoying their evening. Sarah and Emily arrived, their faces aglow with pride for the two men who had worked tirelessly toward their dreams.

"Congratulations! We knew you could do it," Sarah said, wrapping Alex in a heartfelt embrace. Emily followed suit with Mark, her admiration in her eyes.

"Thanks, but tonight's not just about celebrating the exam," Alex said, raising his glass. "It's about appreciating everyone who's supported us, especially you two."

"Here's to dreams, hard work, and the best company we could ask for," Mark toasted, clinking glasses with everyone at the table.

Laughter and stories flowed freely, punctuated by the clink of glasses and the low hum of background music. For a few precious hours, thoughts of exams, studying, and future challenges were set aside. Tonight was about the here and now, the joy of camaraderie, and the simple pleasure of being together.

"Remember when we first walked into the gym and saw you both?" Alex reminisced, a playful twinkle in his eye.

"Who could forget?" Emily replied with a chuckle. "You two looked so determined, we couldn't help but be drawn in."

"Looks like that determination paid off," Sarah added, squeezing Alex's hand affectionately.

As the night wore on, the four friends shared in the warmth of their collective spirit, the kind that only comes from shared struggles and mutual aspirations. They were more than friends; they were allies in the pursuit of something greater, each bringing out the best in the others.

"Whatever happens next," Mark said, his gaze sweeping over the group, "we tackle it together."

"Agreed," Alex nodded, clinking his glass once more. "To the next chapter!"

"To the next chapter," they echoed in unison, a pledge to the future they were building—one full of hope, ambition, and the unwavering support of true friends.

As the evening wound down, the giddy energy that had fueled their laughter and conversation began to mellow into a comfortable quietness. The bar was thinning out, its patrons trickling away into the cool night. The four friends lingered in their cozy corner, reluctant to break the spell of camaraderie that encircled them.

Mark found himself studying Emily's features—the way her eyes sparkled when she laughed, how strands of her hair fell gracefully around her face. He caught her gaze, and for a moment, they shared a silent conversation, an understanding that reached beyond words.

"Hey, Emily," Mark said, his voice low, infused with a seriousness that hadn't been there moments before. She tilted her head, listening intently. "I want to tell you something," he continued, watching as curiosity flickered in her eyes. "But not now. I'll wait for the results in a month first."

Emily's expression softened, a gentle smile playing at the corners of her lips. "Okay, Mark," she replied, her hand reaching across the table to give his a reassuring squeeze. "I can wait."

The unspoken promise hung in the air between them, a clue to the depth of their connection. It was a testament to the journey they had all embarked upon together—a journey not just toward professional success, but personal growth and bonds that would last a lifetime.

"Until then," Mark added, lifting his glass once more, "we celebrate the here and now."

"Here and now," they all agreed, their voices mingling in the warm ambiance of the bar. They raised their glasses in a toast, a symbol of unity and the shared dreams that pulsed like a heartbeat through their friendship.

As they eventually said their goodbyes and stepped out into the brisk night, the stars overhead seemed to twinkle with possibility. In the silence of the walk home, Mark felt a sense of peace. The future was uncertain, yes, but it was theirs to shape—with determination, discipline, and the unwavering support of those who mattered most.

The crisp night air brushed against their faces as Alex and Mark made their way back to their shared apartment, the echoes of laughter from the bar receding behind them. The city was asleep, but their minds raced with anticipation.

"Man, that exam," Alex broke the silence, his breath visible in the cool air. "Do you ever think about what happens if we don't pass this one either?"

Mark's footsteps faltered for a moment before regaining pace. "I try not to dwell on it," he admitted, tucking his hands into his jacket pockets. "We've put in too much work not to hope for the best."

Alex nodded, the streetlights casting long shadows as they moved. "Yeah. It's just the waiting, you know? It's like standing at the edge of a cliff, not knowing if you're going to fly or—"

"Or land on something solid," Mark finished for him, a determined glint in his eye. "We'll land on our feet, Alex. We always do."

They reached their building, the familiar hum of the city enveloping them like an old blanket. Upstairs, the apartment felt empty, yet it brimmed with the silent testament of their dreams—the scattered textbooks, the scribbled notes, the worn flashcards. They were artifacts of their relentless pursuit, and as they settled onto the couch, the weight of their journey pressed upon them.

"Third and last exam," Alex mused aloud, running a hand through his hair. The thought of it was a mountain still to climb, its peak shrouded in the mists of the unknown.

"Yeah," Mark replied, leaning back and staring at the ceiling. "But think about it, once we conquer that... we're there. Licensed pharmacists, here, in Canada. Our dream."

"Exactly." Alex leaned forward, elbows on knees, a flicker of excitement cutting through the fatigue. "This is more than a test, Mark. It's proof that all this—waking up at 5 am, hitting the gym, studying until our eyes burn—it's all worth it."

Mark turned to look at his friend, seeing the same fire that had sparked between them when they first set their ten-year goal. It was a fire fueled by ambition, friendship, and the realization that success was forged from resilience.

"Waiting for the results will be tough," Mark acknowledged. "But remember what you said about discipline being the key?"

Alex smiled faintly, remembering their pact, the foundation upon which they'd built their Canadian lives. "Yeah. Discipline."

"Let's keep that in mind," Mark said, rising from the couch. "No matter what those results say, we go again. We study, we work, we push until we can't anymore—because eventually, we won't have to."

Nodding in agreement, Alex stood as well, a silent vow passing between them. They were more than friends; they were each other's anchor in a sea of uncertainty. And together, they would weather any storm.

"Let's get some sleep," Alex suggested. "Tomorrow, we hit the ground running again. No rest for the wicked, right?"

"Right," Mark confirmed, a smirk lifting the corner of his mouth. "And Alex? We are going to pass. Both the results and the third exam. We've got this."

"Damn right, we do," Alex replied, his voice steady with conviction. As they retired to their respective rooms, the night embraced them in its quiet promise. Tomorrow was another step toward their dreams, and they were ready to take it—together.

After a month of waiting for the results the morning sun filtered through the blinds, casting stripes of light over the two friends huddled around a small kitchen table. Their apartment, usually echoing with the clatter of study materials and determined whispers, was now suffused with an anxious silence.

Alex's hands trembled slightly as he refreshed his email inbox for what felt like the hundredth time that hour. Mark paced behind him, each step a testament to their shared tension. The date had been circled on their calendar, both a beacon and a specter: Results Day.

"Come on," Alex muttered under his breath, his eyes locked on the screen. "Just show up already."

Mark stopped pacing and placed a steadying hand on Alex's shoulder. "It'll be there when it's there," he said, though his voice betrayed his own eagerness for news.

"Easy for you to say," Alex replied with a half-hearted grin. "You're not the one hitting refresh."

"Fine, switch then. I'll hit refresh, and you pace," Mark suggested, trying to inject some levity into the wait.

Before they could swap places, however, the laptop pinged—a sound both mundane and momentous. An email from the Pharmacy Examining Board of Canada sat in Alex's inbox, its subject line glaring back at them: Examination Results.

Their hearts pounded in unison as Alex clicked the message open. Time seemed to slow, the cursor an extension of their collective willpower, urging the contents to reveal themselves.

"Dear Candidate," the email began, and Alex read aloud, "...we are pleased to inform you..."

A cheer erupted between them, the words blurring together as the realization dawned: they had passed.

"YES!" Mark shouted, lifting Alex from his chair and into an impromptu victory dance around the tiny kitchen. "We did it, man! We actually did it!"

"Can you believe it?" Alex exclaimed, his eyes shining with the reflection of a dream realized.

"All those hours, the sacrifices—we made it count."

"Of course I can believe it," Mark said, finally releasing Alex but keeping a firm grip on his friend's shoulders. "We said we'd do it, and we did. We're going to be pharmacists, Alex. This is just the beginning."

"Right, the beginning," Alex repeated, his thoughts already racing ahead. "Now we build, we grow, we—"

"Hey," Mark interrupted gently, "let's just take a moment, okay? Let's appreciate this win. We've earned it."

"Okay," Alex agreed, nodding. He took a deep breath, letting the weight of their achievement settle onto his shoulders—a welcome burden. "We've earned it."

As laughter and plans for the future filled the room, the two stood side by side, emboldened by success and the unshakeable bond that had carried them through. They were more than survivors of the grueling path they had chosen; they were conquerors, ready to claim the lives they had envisioned ten years ago. And nothing would stand in their way.

Mark turned to gaze out the small window above the sink, watching as the sky transformed into a canvas of twilight hues. "But let's not get too carried away," he said. "There's that one last exam looming over us—the final step."

"Right, the third and last one," Alex murmured, his voice a blend of anticipation and resolve. He joined Mark by the window, their reflections merging in the glass. "It's like the final boss in a video game, isn't it? The big baddie at the end of the level."

"Exactly." Mark chuckled. "And just like any epic game, we can't afford to lose focus now. We've come too far to slip up on the home stretch." He glanced at Alex, his expression serious yet confident. "We will do it. Just like we did today."

"Absolutely," Alex agreed. His eyes gleamed with a spirited determination that had been their lodestar since the day they vowed to turn their dreams into reality. He knew the path ahead would demand more from them—more hours of studying, more sacrifices, more unwavering discipline. But the thought didn't scare him. If anything, it steeled his resolve.

"Let's take tonight off, though," Mark suggested, breaking into Alex's thoughts. "Celebrate our victory. Because tomorrow, we go back to war."

"Agreed," Alex said, a smile curving on his lips. "One night to breathe, to live a little. And then we conquer the next challenge."

"Cheers to that," Mark said, raising an imaginary glass. "To us, to our future, and to the final hurdle we're about to clear."

"Cheers," Alex echoed, clinking his own phantom glass against Mark's. Their laughter echoed in the kitchen, light and triumphant—a harbinger of the success they were certain lay just within reach. They had each other, their dreams, and the resilience to face whatever trials awaited them. Together, they were unstoppable.

The next morning, with the triumph of passing still fresh in their spirits but the reality of the upcoming challenge looming, Alex strode over to the bare wall that had been staring at them for too long. The wall needed something—a symbol of their tenacity, a daily reminder that they were on a mission.

"Hey, Mark," Alex called out, his voice bouncing off the kitchen tiles as he rummaged through a drawer. His hand found a marker, and with purpose, he turned to face the empty space beside the door, where every day they would see it before leaving the apartment.

"Watch this." He uncapped the marker with a decisive flick and pressed its tip against the wall. The ink flowed as he scrawled each letter with care, the words growing bold and undeniable: NO SURRENDER.

"Perfect," Mark said, joining him. "It's like our banner, our mantra."

"Exactly," Alex replied, stepping back to admire his handiwork. "We need to see it, live by it. No surrender, no giving up. It's time to make dreams come true."

The black letters stood stark against the white paint, an indelible pledge that resonated within the room. They both knew the power of words, how they could shape thoughts and transform actions. This wasn't just a statement; it was a vow made visible.

"Let's add the rest," Mark suggested, taking the marker from Alex. Below NO SURRENDER, he added, IT'S TIME TO MAKE DREAMS COME TRUE.

They stepped back, side by side, evaluating their creation. It was more than a motto; it was a reflection of their journey, a clue to the unyielding spirit that drove them. Every early morning gym session, every healthy meal, every late night of study—they were all encapsulated in those words on the wall.

"Looks good," Alex said, nodding with satisfaction. His heart swelled with a sense of camaraderie and shared ambition. This board wasn't just about holding onto motivation; it was about honoring the bond that had formed between them, a bond fortified by shared goals and mutual support.

"More than good," Mark replied, a spark of excitement in his eyes. "It looks like victory."

Alex smiled, feeling the weight of their past struggles and the promise of future triumphs. The board on the wall was a testament to their resilience, a declaration that they would not be deterred, no matter the setbacks or the odds.

With renewed vigor, they prepared to step out into the day, under the watchful gaze of their new creed. The journey ahead was clear, and they marched forward, unwavering and resolute, towards the dreams they were determined to turn into their reality.

With the board's affirmation hanging in the air, Alex and Mark strode out of their apartment, the early morning light casting long shadows on the pavement. The crisp breeze seemed to carry with it the freshness of new opportunity, a subtle reminder that each day brought them closer to their aspirations.

"Ready to tell Magie?" Alex asked as they walked side by side.

"Absolutely," Mark responded, his voice steady but laced with an undercurrent of pride. "Passing that second exam was no small feat."

As they entered the pharmacy, the familiar scent of antiseptics and medication greeted them—a scent that now signified more than just their current job; it was the smell of their future profession. They navigated the aisles with purpose until they reached the dispensary, where Magie, the owner, was meticulously organizing prescriptions for the day.

"Magie," Alex called out, garnering her attention.

The woman turned to them, her face etched with lines of experience, eyes sharp behind her glasses. "What is it, boys?" she asked, her tone always hinting at impatience, but not unkindly so.

Mark took the lead, unable to suppress the broad grin spreading across his face. "We passed our second qualifying exam," he announced, the words carrying both relief and triumph.

Magie straightened up, peering at them through her spectacles as if reassessing them in this new light. Her lips twitched into a rare smile, and she laid her hand on a stack of medicine boxes like a queen bestowing a silent benediction upon her knights.

"Well done," she said, the simplicity of her praise belied by the warmth in her gaze. "That's no easy task, especially while working here and keeping your heads in the books."

"Thank you, Magie," Alex chimed in, feeling a swell of gratitude for the woman who had given them a chance, a place to grow and learn even as they worked towards something greater.

"We've still got one more to go," Mark added quickly, eager to show that their ambition hadn't waned with this latest achievement.

"Of course you do," Magie replied, nodding sagely. "And you'll pass that one too. You've got the right attitude—the kind that turns dreams into reality."

Her endorsement filled the room, settling over Alex and Mark like a mantle of responsibility and potential. As they exchanged glances, it was clear that their shared resolve only grew stronger. They were ready to face the final hurdle, to grasp the future that they had been tirelessly sculpting with every disciplined choice and sacrifice.

"Back to work now, boys," Magie instructed, turning back to her duties, her moment of sentimentality tucked away as swiftly as it had appeared.

Alex and Mark nodded and set about their tasks, the routine motions now infused with a fresh sense of purpose. Each customer interaction, each label affixed, each pill counted was a step closer to their goal. And when the day was over, they would return to their studies, fortified by the knowledge that their efforts were not in vain, that their dreams were indeed coming true.

The final customers of the day trickled out of the pharmacy, leaving behind the quiet hum of fluorescent lights and the soft shuffle of Mark's footsteps as he tidied the shelves. Alex was counting the register, his mind already anticipating the evening's study session, when Mark approached him with an unusual hesitance in his gait.

"Hey, Alex," Mark began, his voice betraying a mix of excitement and nerves. "I need to tell you something."

Alex looked up from the cash drawer, meeting his friend's eyes. In them, he saw a familiar fire—one that went beyond exams and career ambitions. It was something deeper, more personal.

"What's up?" Alex asked, closing the drawer with a soft click.

Mark took a deep breath, steadying himself. "I've made a decision. After we close up here, I'm going to meet Emily. And I'm going to tell her... I'm going to tell her that I love her."

The words hung in the air between them, both a declaration and a revelation. Alex straightened up, his expression shifting to one of wholehearted support.

"Man, that's huge," he said, clapping Mark on the shoulder. "You've really fallen for her, huh?"

"More than I thought possible," Mark admitted, a smile breaking across his face. "She's been incredible through all this—through the studying, the stress, the ups and downs. She's more than just a girlfriend; she's a partner in this crazy dream of ours."

Alex nodded in understanding. He had seen the bond between Mark and Emily grow, watched how they rallied around each other, their relationship becoming another cornerstone in the foundation of their shared aspirations.

"Then you should definitely tell her," Alex encouraged. "And hey, no matter what happens, you've got my back, right? Just like with the exams, we're in this together."

"Always," Mark affirmed. With a renewed sense of purpose, he checked his reflection in the small mirror by the door, straightening his pharmacy assistant vest for the last time that day.

"Go get her, man," Alex said with a grin as he turned off the register. "But don't forget—we've still got one more exam to crush."

Mark laughed, the sound light and hopeful. "Wouldn't dream of it. But tonight, I've got a different kind of future to secure."

With a final nod to Alex, Mark stepped out into the cool evening air, his heart buoyant with the possibility of love reciprocated and dreams steadily coming to fruition.

Mark's footsteps echoed with a mix of trepidation and anticipation as he made his way to the small park where he and Emily had agreed to meet. The evening was settling in, painting the sky in hues of dusky pink and orange, a calm backdrop to the storm of emotions whirling inside him.

"Hey," Emily called out, her voice cutting through the silence as she approached from the other side of the fountain that served as their rendezvous point. She wore a light jacket over her casual attire, her hair pulled back in a simple ponytail that accentuated the earnestness in her eyes.

"Hey," Mark replied, trying to steady his nerves. He watched her close the distance between them, each step measured and sure. There was an air of understanding about her that often caught him off guard, a depth that went beyond the surface.

They greeted each with a brief, comfortable hug before sitting side by side on the bench, leaving both space and opening for what was to come. Mark turned to her, the words he had practiced tumbling out in a rush. "Emily, I've been thinking about us—"

She placed a gentle hand on his arm, silencing him with a warm, knowing smile. "Mark, I know what you want to say, and I feel it too. But you told me after you pass the 2nd exam, remember?"

He nodded, the memory clear in his mind. It was one of the countless conversations they'd had amid textbooks and late-night study sessions.

"Then let's wait until after the 3rd exam," she continued, her gaze steady. "I don't want you to be distracted with me. Our dreams are within reach, and I want us both to be able to give them everything we've got."

Mark felt the weight of her words settle in his chest. They were not a dismissal but rather a

commitment to the future they both sought—
one that extended beyond the immediate thrills
of new love. It was a pledge to support each
other unconditionally, even if it meant
postponing personal desires for a greater goal.

"Okay," he said, the corners of his mouth
lifting into a smile that mirrored hers. "After
the 3rd exam, then."

"Promise?" she asked, extending her pinky in a
playful gesture that belied the seriousness of
their pact.

"Promise," Mark confirmed, locking his pinky
with hers. This simple act sealed their
agreement, a symbol of patience and
perseverance that would carry them through
the challenges ahead.

They sat together as evening descended upon
the park, talking softly about everything and
nothing, two hearts beating in sync with a
shared vision of the future. And in that quiet
moment, Mark knew that no matter the
outcome of their next endeavor, they would
face it together, unafraid and undistracted.

Eventually, the sky shifted into twilight hues,
and the air grew cooler around them. Mark
glanced at Emily, noticing the way the fading

light played across her features, casting a serene glow. It was time to head back, yet neither of them seemed eager to break the comfortable silence that had enveloped them.

"Guess we should get going," Mark finally said, his voice low, not wanting to disrupt the tranquility of the moment.

Emily nodded, standing up from the bench where they'd been seated. They walked side by side toward the park's exit, their steps unhurried. The world around them transitioned from the park's natural oasis to the familiar cityscape as they made their way through the streets towards home.

As they approached the doorstep of the apartment complex, they paused, turning to face each other. There was a magnetic pull in the space between them, a connection strengthened by shared goals and mutual respect. Mark stepped forward, enveloping Emily in a warm embrace. She reciprocated, her arms wrapping around him, holding on tightly for a long moment.

"Thanks for understanding, Em," Mark murmured against her hair.

"Always," she whispered back, her voice muffled against his chest.

They lingered in the hug, finding comfort in the assurance of their bond. Eventually, they parted, yet the warmth from their embrace remained, a reminder of the support system they had built together.

"See you tomorrow at the gym?" Mark asked, a hint of playfulness returning to his tone.

"Wouldn't miss it," Emily replied, her smile reaching her eyes. "Goodnight, Mark."

"Goodnight, Emily."

With another final, knowing look shared between them, they turned to their separate doors. As Mark entered his apartment, he felt a renewed sense of purpose. He and Alex had come so far, and with Emily and Sarah by their side, there was a sense that anything was possible.

He closed the door behind him, ready for whatever challenges lay ahead, fortified by the knowledge that love and ambition could coexist, propelling them all toward the futures they dared to dream.

The apartment door closed with a soft click, and Mark leaned back against the wood, exhaling slowly. He could still feel the warmth of Emily's hug lingering on his skin, an echo of the connection that had grown between them over months of shared experiences and mutual encouragement.

"Hey," Alex's voice snapped Mark out of his reverie. His friend was seated at the small kitchen table, surrounded by an array of textbooks and notes, indicative of their relentless pursuit of becoming licensed pharmacists. A look of mild concern etched Alex's features, eyebrows raised in silent inquiry.

Mark pushed off from the door and walked over to join him, pulling out a chair and slumping down with a mixture of fatigue and resolve coloring his posture.

"Everything okay?" Alex asked, eyes searching Mark's face for clues.

Mark nodded, then took a moment to gather his thoughts before diving into the tale of the evening. "Yeah, it went... it went really well, actually." He paused, his lips curving into a half-smile as he recalled Emily's understanding nature. "I told her, y'know, what I've been feeling. About her."

Alex leaned forward, his attention focused entirely on Mark. There was no hint of impatience; only the steady support that had become the cornerstone of their friendship.

"And?" Alex prompted when Mark hesitated, the single word laden with curiosity and brotherly solidarity.

"She said she feels the same," Mark continued, the smile now fully formed as relief washed over him. But then his expression sobered slightly. "But she also said we should wait until after the third exam. She doesn't want us to get distracted, wants us to stay focused."

"Sounds like she really gets it—the dream, the grind, all of it," Alex said, nodding approvingly.

"Yeah, she does." Mark's voice was thick with gratitude. The journey they'd embarked upon was demanding, often a test of endurance as much as intellect, but having someone like Emily in his corner made the sacrifices feel worthwhile.

"Good. We need people who understand the vision, not just the present moment," Alex added, and Mark could hear the unspoken acknowledgment of their own friendship in those words.

"Exactly." Mark let out a contented sigh, finally allowing himself to relax into the chair. "Thanks, man. For asking, for listening—just for being here."

"Always," Alex echoed Emily's earlier sentiment, giving Mark a solid, reassuring pat on the shoulder.

They sat there for a while longer, two friends united by their ambitions and the shared belief that hard work and discipline would eventually pay off. Tomorrow would bring another early morning at the gym, another long day of work and study, but for now, this quiet moment of camaraderie was enough.

"Alright, time to hit the sack. Big day tomorrow," Alex said, standing up and stretching his arms above his head.

"Yep." Mark stood as well, feeling a renewed vigor infuse his limbs. "Let's ace that third exam, build our empire, and never forget why we started."

"Absolutely," Alex agreed, a determined glint in his eye. "No surrender, right?"

"No surrender," Mark affirmed, and together, they turned off the lights and headed to bed, ready to face another day in pursuit of their ten-year dream.

The clinking of weights and the rhythmic thud of running shoes on treadmills filled the gym with the familiar cacophony of exertion. Alex and Mark, side by side, pushed through their morning workout with a silent tenacity that had become as routine as the sunrise.

Mark glanced at Alex, noting the beads of sweat that traced the determined lines of his friend's face. They were in this together— every lift, every mile, every early morning was a step toward their shared goal. The vision of success that pulled them out of bed at 5 AM each day was no less vivid now than it had been when they first dared to dream it.

"Three more reps, come on," Alex grunted, as he steadied the barbell overhead.

"Got it," Mark replied, his muscles burning with the effort but his mind clear and focused. They finished their set and moved onto the next exercise, a silent agreement between them that there would be no compromise, no half-measures.

After the gym, they rode the subway, surrounded by the press of bodies and the soft murmur of commuters starting their day. Mark reviewed flashcards while Alex jotted down notes from a pharmaceutical textbook, both making use of every spare moment. Their dedication was a shield against doubt, a fortress built with the bricks of discipline and ambition.

At work, where they work as a pharmacy assistant . Each interaction was an opportunity to learn, to store away knowledge for the future when they would stand behind their own counters, dispensing not only drugs but the dreams they had worked so hard to realize.

Evenings were reserved for study, the quiet of the apartment punctuated by the rustle of pages and the scratch of pens. They poured over their materials, quizzing each other, challenging each other to reach deeper understandings of complex subjects.

"Remember, it's not just about passing the exam," Alex said, his eyes never leaving the page. "It's about being the best pharmacists we can be—for our patients, for ourselves."

"Right," Mark agreed, the weight of responsibility settling comfortably on his shoulders. This wasn't just about personal gain; it was about the impact they could have, the lives they could change with their knowledge and care.

As midnight approached, they allowed themselves a brief respite, a moment to reflect on the progress made and the journey still ahead. The path was steep, the obstacles many, but Alex and Mark knew that their unwavering commitment to their goals would carry them through.

"Tomorrow, we do it all over again," Mark said, a smile tugging at the corner of his mouth.

"Every day, until we get there," Alex responded, matching his friend's expression with a confident grin of his own.

They turned in for the night, bodies exhausted but spirits undimmed, each challenge faced another clue that they were inching ever closer to the richness of a dream fulfilled.

The next morning arrived with the usual symphony of alarm clocks and groans of reluctance, but Alex and Mark were out of their beds before the echoes faded. They laced up their sneakers, their movements synchronized by routine and shared ambition.

The gym was quiet in the early hours, save for the clanking of weights and the steady hum of treadmills. Alex powered through his reps, each lift a testament to his discipline, while Mark counted off the sets, his voice steady and encouraging. The physical exertion was more than a quest for health; it was a metaphor for their tenacity, the strength required to shoulder their aspirations.

"Discipline," Alex panted between breaths, "is what will make us rich—not just in wealth, but in character."

"Exactly," Mark replied as he adjusted the weight on the barbell. "We're building more than muscle here."

Work awaited them, a reality check against their dreams, but they faced it head-on, carrying the energy from their morning workout into their daily tasks. At the pharmacy, they navigated the shelves and prescriptions with precision, their interactions with customers tinged with the knowledge that they too, would soon be dispensing not just medicine, but advice and compassion as licensed pharmacists.

Night descended, and with it came the return to their books. The apartment, once again, became a sanctuary of study. They quizzed each other on drug interactions and proper dosages, their minds absorbing information that would one day be crucial in someone's care.

"Imagine," Mark said during a brief pause, "when all this studying pays off, and we can truly make a difference."

Alex nodded, his fatigue replaced by a surge of purpose. "Every question we answer correctly could be a life saved. That's the real richness we're chasing."

With that, they delved back into their studies, the late hours passing unnoticed as they fortified their resolve. Each chapter read, each practice question answered, brought them closer to their goal—a goal that extended far beyond financial success and into the realm of impacting human lives for the better.

"Tomorrow," Alex finally said as they prepared to sleep, "we rise, and we conquer again."

"Every day, every night," Mark echoed, "until our dream is no longer a dream."

In the stillness of their room, two friends lay restful yet restless, their shared vision clearer than ever, a beacon guiding them through the darkness toward the dawn of their success.

The pattern of their lives had become a rhythm, a heartbeat pulsing with discipline and ambition. Morning light would filter through the blinds, casting lines of gold across their shared space, a silent signal for the day to begin. With the sound of an alarm breaking the hush of dawn, they would rise in unison, the air charged with determination.

In the gym, weights clanged and treadmills hummed, the echo of their exertion blending into a symphony of effort. They pushed themselves, not just for strength of body but for clarity of mind, each drop of sweat a testament to their unwavering commitment.

"Keep going," Alex would grunt between sets, his muscles burning with the sweet pain of progress.

"Never stop," Mark would reply, spotting his friend, ensuring every rep was a step toward their collective aspiration.

Work was no less grueling, long hours behind the counter, where patience was as necessary as knowledge. But even there, amid the bustle of customers and the scent of freshly counted pills, their dream did not wane. It lived in every interaction, every piece of advice dispensed with a prescription.

"Remember why we're here," Mark would remind Alex during moments of weariness.

"For them, for us," Alex would affirm, his gaze firm on the horizon of their future.

And then the nights, oh, the nights where the world quieted but their minds raced faster than ever. Page after page turned, notes upon notes taken; their apartment became a crucible of learning, each study session forging them closer to readiness.

"Almost there," Alex would say, his voice soft with exhaustion but fierce with hope.

"Almost," Mark would agree, his own eyes heavy but gleaming with the same fire that drove them forward.

This cycle, this relentless pursuit of excellence, continued day after day, month after month. Every sunrise brought them nearer to their goal, every sunset left them more equipped for the challenges ahead. The third and last exam loomed on the horizon like a mountain peak, daunting yet within reach.

Finally, the day arrived. The culmination of all their efforts, all their sacrifices, stood before them, no longer an abstract point in the future but a tangible moment in time. They donned their armor, not of metal and leather, but of knowledge and experience, ready to face their destiny.

"Today, we conquer," Alex said, his voice steady, his heart racing.

"Today," Mark echoed, "we make our dreams reality."

With their heads held high and their spirits unbreakable, they stepped out into the dawn's early light, bound for the exam center. Today, they would not just take a test; they would seize their future with hands ready to heal, ready to serve, ready to embrace the richness of a life lived for others. Today, they would become pharmacists.

The crisp morning air nipped at their faces as they made their way through the quiet streets of Toronto, the city just beginning to stir. The exam center was not far, but each step seemed to carry the weight of their years-long journey.

"Hey," Alex broke the silence, a hint of excitement threading through his voice as they turned a corner. "I had this dream last night."

Mark glanced over, eyebrows raised in curiosity. "Yeah?"

"I dreamed that we passed," Alex confessed, almost breathless with the vividness of the memory. "It felt so real, like I could almost touch the certificate."

"Let's hope it's a good omen," Mark replied, the edges of a smile tugging at his lips. "Dreams have a way of pointing us toward what we want most."

"Exactly," Alex agreed, feeling a surge of confidence. "We've worked too hard to let anything stand in our way now."

They reached the entrance of the exam center, the building imposing yet somehow welcoming. Other exam-takers milled around, some poring over last-minute notes, others simply waiting in quiet anticipation.

Alex and Mark exchanged a look, a silent pact between them. They had faced every challenge together, lifted each other up through moments of doubt, and now they stood on the brink of realizing their shared ambition.

"Ready?" Mark asked, his hand on the door.

"More than ever," Alex replied, nodding resolutely.

Together, they stepped inside, the door closing behind them with a soft click. The future awaited, and they were ready to claim it.

The room was a hive of focused energy as Alex and Mark took their seats among the other candidates. They had been through the rigor of exams before, but this one felt different; it was not just another test, it was the culmination of all their sacrifices, the gateway to the future they had envisioned.

Papers shuffled, pens clicked, and nervous glances were exchanged. The invigilator's voice sliced through the tension, announcing the start of the exam. This was it—the proving ground of their knowledge, skills, and unwavering determination.

Alex picked up his pen, his hand steady as he filled in the necessary details on his paper. He looked up for a moment, meeting Mark's gaze across the room. There was no need for words; their eyes conveyed mutual support and a shared resolve.

As the hours ticked by, Alex found himself absorbed in the questions before him, each one a stepping stone towards his goal. He methodically worked through the scenarios, diagnosing, prescribing, counseling—each action practiced and precise, honed by months of relentless study.

Mark was equally immersed, his focus never wavering as he interacted with the simulated patients, a test designed to measure not only their pharmaceutical knowledge but also their ability to apply it in real-world situations.

They had learned long ago that success hinged on more than just intelligence; it was about empathy, communication, and the ability to make a difference in people's lives—qualities they both strived to embody.

Finally, the invigilator called time, and the spell of concentration was broken. Alex put down his pen, a sense of relief washing over him. He glanced around the room, seeing the same exhaustion and hope reflected in the faces of his peers.

The two friends met outside the examination hall, a silent understanding passing between them. They had given it their all, left nothing in reserve. Now, all they could do was wait for the results that would seal their fate.

"Whatever happens," Mark said, breaking the quiet that had settled between them, "we've already won."

Alex nodded, feeling a smile creep onto his face despite the lingering nerves. "We've come this far together. We're not just dreamers anymore—we're doers."

As they walked away from the exam center, Alex couldn't help but think back to his dream, the vivid sensation of success. Maybe it was more than just a dream; perhaps it was a premonition. Whatever it was, Alex knew one thing for sure: together with Mark, he was ready to turn that dream into reality.

Days passed, each one stretching longer than the last as Alex and Mark's anxiety grew. They tried to maintain their routine—gym, work, study—but the weight of anticipation hung heavy in their shared apartment, thickening the air with tension.

"Remember, it's out of our hands now," Mark would often say, trying to instill a sense of calm, but his own restless energy betrayed him.

They distracted themselves with plans for the future, discussing business ideas and investment strategies, yet their thoughts inevitably circled back to the looming verdict of their exams.

Then, on a Tuesday that had begun like any other, with the pale light of dawn seeping into their living room, Alex's phone pinged with an alert. Heart hammering against his ribs, he fumbled to unlock the screen.

"Mark!" he shouted, voice cracking in a blend of hope and dread. "It's here!"

Mark bolted from the kitchen, nearly tripping over a chair in his haste. Together they hunched over the glowing screen, shoulder to shoulder, eyes scanning the email that held their future.

"Congratulations..." Alex read aloud, the word barely a whisper, but it was enough.

A moment of stunned silence enveloped them before reality set in, and then, suddenly, the room erupted with their elated roars. They jumped around like lottery winners, arms flailing, voices climbing octaves in unbridled joy.

"We did it, man! We freaking did it!" Alex whooped, his dreams validated by those few, precious words.

"Pharmacists! Can you believe it?" Mark added, laughter and tears mingling on his face.

In the midst of their celebration, they clasped hands, a pact of brotherhood stronger than ever. This victory wasn't just a personal triumph; it was a shared conquest, the culmination of countless hours of shared sacrifice and determination.

"Simon won't believe this," Alex managed to say between shouts, thinking of their supportive friend who had always believed in them.

"Let's call him! Let's call everyone!" Mark suggested, already reaching for his phone.

Their journey had been arduous, filled with obstacles and doubts, but as they stood there, reveling in their success, it all seemed worth it. The future stretched out before them, bright and inviting, a blank canvas ready to be painted with the colors of their ambition.

And in that moment, Alex knew that no matter what challenges lay ahead, they were ready to face them together.

Alex grabbed his own phone, its screen smeared with the evidence of their earlier tension. His fingers danced over the buttons with a frenzied urgency, the need to share the news burning like fire in his chest.

"Emily first or Sarah?" Alex asked, his voice brimming with excitement as he looked at Mark.

"Call them both, conference style!" Mark suggested, the grin on his face stretching from ear to ear.

With a few swift taps, Alex merged the calls and put the phone on speaker. The ringing seemed to echo the rapid beating of their hearts—each tone heightening the anticipation until finally, a click signaled connection.

"Sarah? Emily? We've got some incredible news!" Alex burst out before the girls could even offer greetings.

"Hey guys! What's up? You sound... ecstatic," came Sarah's voice, warm and curious.

"Tell us everything!" Emily chimed in, her voice carrying the smile that was surely on her face.

"We passed, we're officially qualified pharmacists!" Mark exclaimed, unable to keep the pride out of his voice.

The squeals from the other end of the line were music to their ears, another sweet confirmation of their success.

"Congratulations, you two! We knew you could do it!" Sarah cheered, her voice a melodious symphony to their ears.

"Let's celebrate! When are we seeing you?" Emily added, laughter and joy weaving through her words.

"Tonight. Let's meet tonight and make it unforgettable!" Mark said, already thinking of places to go.

"Absolutely! This is the best news ever!" Emily agreed wholeheartedly.

"Guys, I can't even express how happy I am right now," Alex confessed, his voice trembling slightly with the magnitude of their achievement.

"Neither can we," Mark added, glancing at Alex with a wide, triumphant smile. "It's like we're dreaming."

"Then let's not wake up from this dream just yet," Sarah said, her tone playful and uplifting.

"See you tonight, heroes!" Emily concluded, before they said their goodbyes, each promise of celebration like a vow for continued support and shared dreams.

As the call ended, Alex and Mark looked at each other, the weight of their accomplishment sinking in. They had climbed the mountain, faced the trials, and now, the horizon was theirs to explore. Their relentless spirit, once tested by failures and fears, now soared high on the wings of victory.

The crisp evening air brushed against Alex and Mark's faces as they pushed open the door to the local bar, the familiar clamor of patrons and clinking glasses wrapping around them like a welcome home. They scanned the crowd, eyes searching for the two beacons who had become their pillars of strength in recent times.

"Over here!" The shout came from Sarah, her arm waving energetically above the heads of merrymakers.

Alex caught her eye and felt an immediate rush of warmth. Beside Sarah, Emily stood with an equally excited grin. Their eyes sparkled with pride and anticipation, reflecting the dim lighting of the bar like stars brought down to earth. Mark locked eyes with Emily, and his heart skipped a beat at the sight of her joyous expression.

With swift strides cutting through the bustling crowd, Alex and Mark approached the table. Without hesitation, they were wrapped in an embrace that melded four souls into one triumphant force. The hug was a physical manifestation of shared struggles and collective dreams; it was tight and full of meaning, speaking volumes without a single word.

"Look at you two, all certified and official now!" Emily exclaimed as they finally pulled away, her eyes shining with admiration.

"Let's toast to determination and dreams that refuse to die," Sarah suggested, raising her glass high.

Glasses were raised, clinking in a chorus of hope and achievement. The bubbly liquid fizzed on their tongues, but it was nothing compared to the effervescent joy bubbling in their chests. Laughter erupted from their small circle, each chuckle a note in the symphony of their shared journey.

"Here's to new beginnings," Alex announced, his voice steady and sure.

"To love and support that sees us through," Mark added, glancing between the girls and his best friend.

"And to never forgetting why we started," they said in unison, their bond unbreakable.

The night unfolded like a tapestry woven with threads of camaraderie and celebration. Each laugh, each story shared, each glance exchanged under the dim lights of the bar only served to reinforce the unity between them. Tonight, they were not just two friends who wanted to be rich in ten years—they were visionaries on the cusp of greatness, surrounded by those who believed in them unequivocally.

The hours slipped by, unnoticed and swift, as they reminisced over past struggles and toasted to future triumphs. The music pulsed through the bar, a rhythmic heartbeat to their own elevated spirits. Mark caught Emily's eye from across the table, her smile a beacon in the dimly lit space.

"Hey, Emily," Mark called out over the din of celebration, his voice tinged with a nervous excitement that made his heart race.

Emily turned toward him, her face the picture of curiosity overlaid with a hint of something deeper. "Yes?" she responded, leaning in slightly to hear him better.

"Do you remember?" he asked, the moment hanging between them like a clue to a puzzle only they could piece together.

"Remember what?" Her cheeks flushed a delicate shade of pink, the color deepening under the warm glow of the bar lights.

Mark took a deep breath, feeling the weight of the words he was about to utter. This was no mere confession; it was the culmination of countless shared glances and unspoken promises. It was a testament to the bond that had grown between them—strong and undeniable.

"I love you," he said simply, yet with an intensity that caused a hush to fall around their corner of the bar.

Emily's eyes widened, her lips parting in a silent gasp as the redness of her cheeks bloomed further. For a moment, the world seemed to pause, the clamor of the bar fading away into nothingness, leaving only the truth of his declaration hanging in the air.

Then, slowly, her surprise melted into a radiant smile, one that spoke of reciprocated feelings and hopes for a future filled with possibilities. She reached across the table, taking Mark's hand in hers, her fingers warm and reassuring.

"Thank you, Mark," she whispered, her voice a melody that danced straight into his heart. "I've been waiting to hear those words."

And in that instant, amidst the revelry of their hard-earned success, Mark knew that true richness lay not just in the pursuit of wealth or accolades, but in the connections formed along the way—in the unwavering support of friends, the promise of love, and the discipline to chase every dream, no matter the odds.

Mark's hand tightened around Emily's, his pulse quickening at her touch. The ambient noise of the bar surged back into focus, but it was as if they were in their own private universe where nothing could breach the intimacy of this moment.

"Emily," he said, his voice a mix of wonder and affirmation, "I've felt this for so long, and now, to hear you say it too—it means everything."

She leaned forward, her gaze locked with his, a smile playing on her lips that held the promise of a thousand shared tomorrows. "I love you too, Mark. I've been scared to admit it—scared it might distract you, or change things between us. But tonight, seeing you succeed, knowing we're on this journey together, I can't hide it anymore."

The honesty in her eyes, the soft cadence of her confession, it anchored Mark to the spot. All the struggles, the late-night study sessions, the uncertainty of their exams—all of it had led to this point, this perfect juncture where aspirations and emotions collided.

"Nothing will distract me more than not having you by my side," he replied earnestly. "You, Sarah, Alex—we're a team. And no exam, no challenge, is greater than what we can overcome together."

Laughter and music swirled around them, but the revelry paled in comparison to the joy bubbling inside Mark. They had conquered academic trials and professional hurdles, but this—this was the beginning of a more personal journey, one that promised an even greater reward.

Around them, glasses clinked, people cheered, but the clamor became a mere backdrop to the symphony of their hearts beating in unison. In the midst of celebration, in the glow of success and the warmth of affection, Mark and Emily found a new chapter unfolding—a tale of love woven seamlessly into their shared dreams of riches and fulfillment.

The elation of the evening buzzed through Alex as he watched his best friend and Emily share a moment that seemed to encapsulate all their hard work and dedication. He couldn't help but feel a surge of pride for Mark and an overwhelming sense of camaraderie. They had both pushed through, side by side, transforming their lives from mere pharmacists to potential masters of their destiny.

As the laughter and chatter around them reached a crescendo, Alex leaned forward, capturing the attention of the group with a gentle clearing of his throat. The smile on his face was one of triumph tinged with the gravity of realism.

"Guys," Alex began, his voice steady yet filled with the fervor of their shared dreams, "this is incredible, and we've come so far. We're almost there—almost at the point where we can call ourselves pharmacists without any qualifiers."

He paused, looking around at the faces of those who mattered most—Mark, Emily, Sarah—all brimming with anticipation for the future they were building together.

"But," he continued, tempering the excitement with a note of caution, "we have to remember that there are a couple more months ahead of us. We've got procedures to follow, red tape to navigate before we can officially get our licenses."

The reality of Alex's words settled over the group like a soft blanket, not smothering their joy, but reminding them of the journey still ahead. It was a path they were now well-equipped to travel, fortified by their love for each other and the unwavering support that had become the cornerstone of their relationships.

"We've beaten the exams, we've proven we have what it takes. Now, it's just a matter of time and patience before we can apply for jobs as pharmacists—real pharmacists—and start building the wealth we've dreamed of for so long," Alex concluded, his eyes gleaming with determination and hope.

A murmur of agreement rippled through their small gathering as they took a collective breath, readying themselves for the next phase. The road to riches was never promised to be easy, but with their unyielding spirit and the bonds that tied them so closely, Alex knew they were destined to achieve everything they had set out to do.

And with that, the night carried on, their celebration a brilliant prelude to the many successes that surely lay ahead.

Mark glanced around at the familiar faces, their features illuminated by the dim glow of the bar lights. They were a testament to perseverance, a small circle that had grown immeasurably close through shared struggle and ambition. He raised his glass, catching Emily's eye as he did so, her smile a beacon of warmth in the semi-darkness.

"Friends," Mark began, his voice steady despite the swell of emotions, "this is just the beginning of our way. We spent the last two years with our noses buried in books, juggling work at Tim Hortons, and pushing through every challenge thrown at us."

He paused, looking at each of them in turn—Alex, with his relentless drive; Sarah, whose encouragement never waned; and Emily, whose belief in him had become his anchor.

"We are pharmacists now," he continued, the title rolling off his tongue with a mixture of pride and awe. "Not just in name, but in spirit. We've earned this. And yes, there's more to do before we can practice, but think about how far we've come."

A collective nod passed among them, a silent acknowledgment of the hurdles they'd overcome and the unwavering dedication that had brought them to this precipice of their future.

"Tomorrow, next month, next year—they're all steps on the path we chose. Steps towards the richness of life we've envisioned. And I don't just mean money in our pockets, but the wealth of experiences, the bonds we've forged, and the lives we'll impact."

He lowered his glass, his gaze locking with each of theirs, conveying an unspoken vow—a promise to continue chasing their dreams, no matter what lay ahead.

"Here's to the journey," Mark said with a smile. "To the late nights, the early mornings, the exams, and the victories. Our dreams are within reach. Let's go out there and live them."

The night air was cool as they eventually stepped outside, the stars overhead bearing witness to their resolve. As they went their separate ways, the excitement of the evening lingered, a prelude to the new chapter that awaited them. The path would be long, undoubtedly filled with more tests and trials, but Mark knew one thing for certain—they were ready.

The cool morning air brushed against Alex's skin as he laced up his running shoes, the sun barely peeking over the horizon. The city was quiet, the usual hum of traffic and life not yet begun. This tranquility was a stark contrast to the celebratory atmosphere from the night before, but it suited Alex's reflective mood.

"New chapter, eh?" Mark mumbled sleepily, stretching his limbs and fighting off the last tendrils of slumber.

"Exactly," Alex replied, standing up and taking a deep breath. He felt the weight of textbooks and study guides lift from his shoulders, replaced by an intangible sense of possibility.

"No more studying. Now we start investing in our future in a different way."

They stepped out into the crisp morning, their footsteps steady on the pavement as they jogged towards the gym. The rhythm of their stride became a meditation, syncing with the pulse of the waking city around them.

"Once we're working as pharmacists, we'll have a bit more financial freedom. We need to be smart with it," Alex continued, his breaths measured despite the exertion. "We save some, sure, but we also need to grow what we earn."

Mark nodded, following Alex's train of thought. "Investing, right? Stocks, real estate – that kind of thing?"

"Exactly. We've spent years learning the chemistry of medicines; now it's time to learn the chemistry of money. How it works, how it grows. Compound interest, passive income – these are going to be our new vocabulary."

Their sneakers thudded against the rubber mat as they entered the gym, the familiar scent of effort and determination greeting them. As they began their workout, each lift and press wasn't just about physical strength; it was symbolic of their commitment to building their future, rep by determined rep.

"First things first, though," Mark said between sets, a grin spreading across his face. "We get our licenses, we secure jobs, then we can dive headfirst into the world of investing."

"Right," Alex agreed, clapping Mark on the back. "And until then, we keep pushing forward, just like always."

The clang of weights punctuated their conversation, a soundtrack to their resilience. They had come this far by supporting one another, by sharing dreams and shouldering burdens together. And as they moved through their workout routine, it was clear that no matter what challenges or opportunities lay ahead, they would face them side by side.

The gym session concluded with their customary fist bump, a silent pact of camaraderie and shared purpose. They exited the building, the early morning sun casting long shadows on the pavement. Alex felt the familiar pull of anticipation for the day ahead, knowing each task was another step toward their grand ambition.

"Remember, we're on shift together today," Mark reminded him as they approached the pharmacy, the sign above the door shining in the bright light.

"Wouldn't miss it," Alex replied, his mind already flipping through the mental checklist of duties that awaited them. He held the door open for Mark, and they stepped into the cool, antiseptic air of the pharmacy.

The workday unfurled with the usual rhythm: counting pills, labeling bottles, consulting with patients. Alex's hands moved with practiced ease, but his thoughts were often elsewhere – on the horizon of their dreams.

"Hey, Alex!" Maggie called out from behind the counter, her voice cutting through his reverie. "Could you help Mrs. Henderson with her prescription? She has questions about her new medication."

"Of course, Maggie," he responded, offering the elderly customer a reassuring smile. As he explained the dosage instructions, his clear communication and genuine concern for her well-being reflected his readiness for more than just the tasks of an assistant.

"Thank you, dear," Mrs. Henderson said, clutching her medicine close. "You young men are going to make fine pharmacists one day."

"Thank you, Mrs. Henderson. That means a lot," Alex replied, pride swelling within him. It was small moments like these that reinforced their purpose, reminding them that their aspirations weren't just about wealth; they were about making a difference.

The day passed in a blur of activity, and as the closing hour neared, Alex found himself tidying up the shelves, aligning boxes and containers with meticulous care. Mark joined him, and together they worked in comfortable silence until the last customer had departed and the doors were locked.

"Alright," Mark said, clapping his hands together as they hung up their white coats. "Ready for that talk?"

"Definitely," Alex replied with a nod, feeling a mixture of excitement and nerves at the prospect of initiating their next phase. "Let's head home and lay it all out. Budgets, plans, research – we'll tackle it all."

"Agreed," Mark said. "And remember, whatever happens, we've got each other's backs."

"Always," Alex affirmed, and they left the pharmacy, the evening air fresh against their faces. The walk back to their apartment was filled with casual banter, but underneath the light-hearted exchange, there was a palpable sense of determination.

They arrived at their modest dwelling, a sanctuary of sorts where countless study sessions and strategy talks had taken place. As they settled into the worn couch, laptops at the ready, Alex couldn't help but feel that this night would mark the beginning of something extraordinary. With a shared glance, they dove into the world of financial education, each link clicked and article read forging the first links in the chain of their envisioned empire.

"Let's make our ten-year promise a reality," Alex said, his voice steady with resolve.

"Ten years to rich," Mark echoed, his eyes bright with the prospect of the future.

Together, they began to build the blueprint of their dreams.

The room was silent except for the occasional click of a mouse or a soft sigh as they delved into the depths of business planning. On the couch, amidst cushioned forts of financial textbooks and dog-eared notebooks, Alex leaned forward, his gaze fixed on the glowing screen before him. Mark mirrored his posture, his own focus unwavering.

"Okay, so," Alex started, breaking the silence, "we've got to be smart about this. We need a solid savings plan if we're going to bootstrap our own pharmacy." He paused, running a hand through his hair, a gesture that had become familiar in times of deep thought.

"Right," Mark agreed, tapping a rhythmic pattern on the keyboard as he pulled up a budget spreadsheet. "We'll cut back where we can, maybe pick up some extra shifts. But we have to keep our end goal in sight."

"Exactly. And it's not just about saving; it's about investing wisely," Alex continued, his voice laced with the enthusiasm of their shared ambition. "We can't just let our money sit there. It needs to work for us."

"Compound interest is our best friend," Mark added with a wry smile, referring to their recent foray into the world of finance.

"True," Alex replied with a chuckle. "But remember, the independent pharmacy is just the first step. Once we're established, we expand, diversify. Maybe even look into developing our own product line someday."

"Getting ahead of ourselves, aren't we?" Mark teased, yet the sparkle in his eye told Alex they were both equally captivated by the grandeur of their dreams.

"Maybe," Alex conceded with a grin, "but why not? Dream big or go home, right?"

"Always dream big," Mark affirmed. "Let's get these numbers crunched. We're on the brink of something huge, my friend."

"Agreed. Let's make sure we're ready for it," Alex said, his fingers dancing over the keys as he began to outline their financial roadmap.

Their conversation drifted into the night, from savings strategies to potential locations, each idea building upon the last like the pieces of an intricate puzzle. They were two friends, united by ambition, fueled by a promise, and on the cusp of turning their shared vision of wealth and success into reality.

The crisp morning air greeted Alex and Mark as they strode purposefully down the tree-lined street toward the pharmacy. The familiar scent of fresh blooms from the surrounding gardens invigorated their spirits, silently reminding them of new beginnings and growth.

"Morning joggers are out in full force today," Mark remarked, noting the steady stream of runners on the opposite sidewalk, each lost in their own rhythm.

"Seems like everyone's chasing their form of success." Alex nodded thoughtfully, adjusting his backpack strap. "Makes you appreciate our own hustle."

"Absolutely. Every step we take is one closer to—"

"Boys!" The sudden call cut through their conversation. They stopped and turned to see Magie, the owner of the pharmacy where they were assisting, emerging from her car with a warm smile that crinkled the corners of her eyes.

"Good morning, Magie," they chorused, matching her friendly tone.

"Good morning indeed! I've been meaning to chat with you both," she said, locking her car before walking briskly over to them. Her gray hair was neatly tied back, revealing the sharp intelligence in her gaze—a gaze that had witnessed decades of community service.

Alex and Mark exchanged a glance, curiosity piqued. Magie wasn't one for small talk during work hours, which meant this had to be important.

"Listen up," she said, clasping her hands together. "I've seen how hard you boys have been working—not just here, but towards your licenses too. It's impressive, really."

"Thank you, Magie," Mark replied. "We're doing our best."

"That's clear as day, and it got me thinking," she continued, her eyes flicking between them. "Once you get your licenses, I want to offer you positions here. Not as assistants, mind you, but as pharmacists."

Alex felt a jolt of excitement surge through him. This was it—the opportunity they had been working towards, the validation of their efforts, the first real step into their future careers.

"Really?" His voice was a mix of surprise and gratitude.

"Absolutely," Magie affirmed with a decisive nod. "You've both got sharp minds and good hearts. That's what this community needs, and that's what I want in my pharmacy."

"Magie, that means the world to us," Mark said, the sincerity in his tone matching the gratitude in Alex's chest. "We won't let you down."

"I know you won't," she said confidently. "Now, let's get inside. There's much to do, and not a moment to waste!"

As they followed Magie into the pharmacy, the early morning conversation about their financial plans seemed like a distant echo. Here was a tangible piece of their dream falling into place, a clue that their ten-year goal was not only attainable but well within reach.

They stepped through the door, ready to embrace the day's challenges, fortified by the promise of a bright and prosperous future.

The day at the pharmacy was a marathon of activity—filling prescriptions, consulting with patients, and navigating the ins and outs of pharmaceutical care under Magie's watchful eye. The energy in the air was palpable, each task another rung on the ladder they were rapidly ascending.

Hours later, as the sun dipped below the horizon, painting the sky in shades of orange and purple, Alex and Mark locked the pharmacy door behind them, their bodies weary but spirits undiminished. They had proven their mettle to Magie, and to themselves.

"Man, that was intense," Alex sighed, rolling his shoulders to ease the tension.

"Good intense," Mark countered, a tired smile spreading across his face. "Feels like we're actually doing it, you know?"

"Totally," Alex agreed, his fatigue momentarily forgotten. "But now, we've got another mountain to climb."

Mark nodded. The promise of future success was exhilarating, but they both understood that dreams didn't manifest from desire alone. It took knowledge, planning, and the wisdom to navigate the financial landscapes that lay before them.

The apartment was quiet when they arrived, a blank canvas awaiting their next moves. Alex powered up his laptop while Mark arranged a stack of notes and textbooks on the coffee table. They settled into their familiar routine, this time not with medical texts but with financial tutorials and investment strategies spread out before them.

"Okay," Alex began, his eyes scanning the screen for the online course they had enrolled in. "Module one: 'Understanding the Stock Market.' Ready?"

"Let's do it," Mark confirmed, leaning forward with keen interest. "We're not just going to be pharmacists, Alex. We're going to be savvy business owners, too."

"Exactly," Alex said, clicking play on the introductory video. "And every bit of knowledge we gain is going to be a piece of our future empire."

Their minds, so adept at absorbing complex medical information, now turned to P/E ratios, market trends, and the intricacies of asset allocation. They shared a mutual hunger to learn, their ambitions fueling late-night study sessions that transcended their immediate goals.

"Think about it," Mark mused during a pause, stretching his legs out. "When we have our own pharmacy, we'll be in control. Not just of our careers, but of our financial destinies, too."

"Exactly," Alex echoed, his voice resolute. "We're building something that lasts, something that goes beyond us. Wealth that'll make a difference—not just for us, but for our community."

They pushed on through the night, the glow from the laptop casting long shadows across the room. Their dreams were not diminished by the setbacks faced or the hard work required. Instead, they were emboldened, the vision of wealth and impact clearer with each passing hour.

As dawn approached, they finally closed their books, a sense of accomplishment settling over them. In the quiet before the city awoke, they shared a look of understanding. This was more than preparation; this was a pledge—a commitment to their future, and to the unbreakable bond that would lead them there.

The sun peeked through the curtains of their spartan living room, casting a soft light on the two friends. They stood and stretched, weary from the night's endeavors yet invigorated by the thought of what lay ahead.

"Remember when we thought about getting that old sedan?" Alex said with a chuckle as he glanced out the window at the bustling street below, where cars zoomed past in the early morning rush.

"Good thing we didn't," Mark replied, his voice laced with a sense of pride. "Every dollar we didn't spend is a brick in the foundation of our pharmacy."

"True," Alex agreed, nodding. He walked over to a jar sitting on the kitchen counter, filled with coins and crumpled bills—their makeshift savings for the dream they both shared. He dropped a few more dollars into it before screwing the lid back on tightly. It was a small gesture, but each contribution was a testament to their dedication.

"Every investment book says the same thing," Mark said, grabbing his water bottle and taking a swig. "It's not just about making money; it's about making smart decisions, living frugally now so we can live abundantly later."

"Like Warren Buffett," Alex mused, his eyes lighting up. "Live like no one else now, so later we can live—and give—like no one else."

"Exactly." Mark smiled, his thoughts already turning to the day ahead. "Alright, let's hit the gym, then head to work. We've got lives to change, remember?"

"Wouldn't miss it for the world," Alex responded, his tone resolute.

They grabbed their gym bags and headed out the door, leaving behind the warmth of their apartment for the crisp, cool air outside. As they walked down the street, side by side, there was a palpable sense of anticipation between them. They knew the road ahead would be long and challenging, but together, they were unstoppable.

Every step they took was a step closer to their dream—a dream they were building with their own two hands, one saved dollar at a time.

Alex felt the familiar rush of adrenaline as they entered the gym. The clang of weights and the rhythmic whir of treadmills were a symphony to his ears—the sound of progress, of potential. He glanced at Mark, who was already warming up, his face set in determination.

"Today's the day," Alex said. "We've been planning, saving, and learning for two years straight. It's time we started looking for locations."

Mark nodded, finishing his last stretch. "I've been crunching numbers all night. We have enough for a down payment on a small place. We just need to find the right spot."

"Location is key," Alex agreed, rotating his shoulders. "We need foot traffic, accessibility, a community that trusts and needs us."

"Let's make a list of potential neighborhoods after our shift at the pharmacy today," Mark suggested, picking up a pair of dumbbells. "We can scout them out this weekend."

"Sounds like a plan," Alex replied, feeling a surge of excitement. All the sacrifices, the long nights studying, the extra shifts, the financial courses—they were all culminating into this moment.

The workout passed in a blur of motion and focus. Each lift, each press, each bead of sweat was symbolic of their unwavering commitment not only to their physical health but also to their shared vision. They pushed each other, driving past the burn, using it as fuel.

Afterward, still catching their breaths, they made their way to the pharmacy. The familiar scent of antiseptics and the sight of neatly lined shelves greeted them, grounding Alex in the reality of what was soon to come. They were on the brink of stepping out from behind these counters and into their own enterprise.

"Hey, boys," Maggie called out from behind the register, her voice carrying over the quiet hum of the store. "How's the big plan coming along?"

"Better than ever, Maggie," Mark answered with a grin. "We're actually going to start looking at places soon."

"Good for you two," she said, her eyes softening with pride. "You're hard workers. You'll make fine pharmacists running your own place."

"Thanks, Maggie," Alex said, warmth spreading through his chest. "That means a lot."

As the day wore on, between advising customers and managing prescriptions, the dream that had once seemed so distant was now within reach. They finished their shift with a sense of accomplishment, eager to dive into the next phase of their journey.

Once home, they unfurled maps and spread out lists, their fingers tracing over areas, marking potential spots. They debated pros and cons, demographics, and competition, every decision scrutinized and deliberate.

"This one looks promising," Alex pointed to a spot on the map, a vibrant area known for its community spirit. "It's near a school and a retirement home. A perfect mix for clientele."

"Let's check it out first thing Saturday," Mark suggested.

"Deal." Alex's heart raced with anticipation. This was it. The culmination of their hard work was finally materializing into something tangible.

"Two years," he murmured, almost to himself. "Two years of grinding, and we're finally here."

"Here and ready to start," Mark echoed, a smile tugging at the corner of his lips.

They sat back, allowing the weight of the moment to settle over them. The path had been far from easy, but they had traversed it together, their friendship and dreams interwoven into a tapestry of ambition and resilience. Now, on the cusp of realizing those dreams, Alex knew that every choice they had made along the way was about to pay off.

The next Saturday, Alex and Mark stood outside the modest storefront that would soon bear their name. The building needed work, but the bones were good – solid, like the foundation of their friendship and shared dreams.

"Alex, picture it," Mark said, his eyes alight with vision. "Our sign right there, clean lines, modern. It'll stand out."

Alex nodded, already visualizing customers walking in, greeted by their friendly staff and the comforting scent of medicine mixed with a hint of hand sanitizer—a beacon of health in the neighborhood.

They shook hands with the real estate agent, the keys heavy and significant in Alex's palm. This was more than just a metal object; it was the key to their future.

"Let's get to work," he said, determination lacing his words.

In the weeks that followed, they painted, shelved, and organized. They interviewed and hired a few employees, imparting the importance of community and care—values at the heart of their business.

"Remember, we're not just pharmacists. We're part of their lives," Alex would say, a mantra for their fledgling enterprise.

Mark took charge of the financials, stretching every dollar, ensuring they remained thrifty without compromising on quality. "Every cent saved is a step closer to our own place," he'd remind Alex when they debated over expenses.

The grand opening day arrived with little fanfare but much significance. The sign above the door gleamed, 'Alex & Mark's Pharmacy,' simple and proud. They welcomed their first customer, an elderly gentleman with a warm smile and a prescription for blood pressure medication.

"Thank you, young men. I've been needing a pharmacy closer to home," he said, his gratitude apparent.

As the man left, Alex caught Mark's eye, a silent exchange passing between them. This was why they had worked tirelessly, why they had studied, scrimped, and saved. The sense of purpose was palpable, as tangible as the pills and potions lining their shelves.

"Here's to us, Alex," Mark said, his voice steady with pride. "To dreams, determination, and doing this together."

"Here's to us," Alex echoed, a smile spreading across his face. They had built something from nothing, fueled by friendship and a promise made long ago.

The bell above the door jingled again, another customer entering. Alex and Mark stepped forward, ready to serve, to heal, and to grow. This pharmacy was more than a business; it was a testament to their journey, a symbol of what two friends could achieve when they dared to dream—and work—as one.

The chime of the bell cut through the hum of activity as Sarah and Emily entered the pharmacy, their arrival infusing the space with a new energy. Alex's eyes lit up at the sight of his wife, a woman whose strength had become the bedrock upon which he could build his aspirations.

"Hey, you made it!" Alex greeted Sarah warmly, crossing the floor with a few eager strides. Sarah's smile was radiant, reflecting the pride she felt for her husband's accomplishments.

"Wouldn't miss it for the world," she replied, reaching out to gently squeeze his hand, a silent message of support passing between them.

Mark looked over from where he was organizing a shelf, his attention captured by Emily's presence. Her encouraging nod was all he needed to reaffirm the path they were on—a path of shared dreams and mutual goals, now intertwined with love and companionship.

"Looks like all that hard work paid off, huh?" Emily said, taking in the neatly arranged displays and the clean, welcoming interior of the pharmacy.

"Every single late night," Mark responded, stepping closer to share a quick, but meaningful hug with Emily.

"Your dedication is inspiring," Sarah added, her gaze sweeping across the store before resting back on Alex. "This place is more than just a business. It's a piece of who you two are."

"Thanks," Alex said, his voice tinged with emotion. "And we couldn't have done it without you both. You're part of this dream, every step of the way."

Sarah and Emily exchanged looks, a shared understanding between them. They had seen their husbands grapple with challenges, buoy each other's spirits during moments of doubt, and now, triumph in the face of adversity.

"Let's make sure this place becomes a cornerstone of the community," Emily suggested, her entrepreneurial spirit shining through.

"Absolutely," Mark agreed. "We're not just here to dispense medication. We're here to care for people, to be a part of their lives."

As customers continued to trickle in, Sarah and Emily stepped aside, allowing Alex and Mark to attend to their needs. Observing them in action, the women saw not just pharmacists, but men of ambition and compassion, husbands they loved and champions of a dream realized.

The day continued, an ebb and flow of patrons and well-wishers, but throughout it all, Alex and Mark never forgot the reason behind their success: a promise, a bond, and two extraordinary women who stood beside them, believing in them when they needed it most.

Amidst the symphony of soft chimes above the door and the occasional crinkle of prescription bags, Alex noticed Sarah's gaze resting thoughtfully on him. The afternoon sunlight filtered through the storefront windows, casting a warm glow over the neatly arranged shelves of medications and health products. Mark, standing behind the counter, was explaining a prescription to an elderly lady with a gentle patience that spoke volumes about his dedication.

"Hey," Sarah said softly once the customer had left, drawing their attention. Her eyes gleamed with a mixture of pride and affection as she looked between Alex and Mark. "The best man to get in love with is one who is ambitious and wants to be better for himself and his family. And we are so proud of you guys."

Her words hung in the air, simple yet profound, encapsulating years of struggle and success into a single sentence. It wasn't just their ambition that Sarah was highlighting; it was their drive to improve not only their own lives but also the lives of those around them.

Mark met her gaze, a slow smile spreading across his face. He reached out, taking Emily's hand and squeezing it gently, gratitude written all over his expression. They had both found partners who didn't merely endure their dreams but actively participated in them.

Alex felt a warmth in his chest that had little to do with the sun's rays. It was the heat of accomplishment, of shared victories, and of love—a love that had proven itself through thick and thin. He crossed the room to where Sarah stood, wrapping an arm around her shoulders and pulling her close.

"Thank you," he murmured, looking into her eyes. "For everything."

Sarah smiled up at him, her head tilting against his embrace. In that moment, surrounded by the tangible evidence of their hard work and the intangible bonds of partnership and mutual support, Alex knew that their journey had only just begun.

The pharmacy door chimed its farewell as Sarah and Emily stepped out, leaving a silence in their wake that was filled with possibility. Alex watched through the glass as they moved down the sidewalk, their laughter echoing back to him. He turned to Mark, whose eyes still lingered on the door, a smile curving his lips.

"Mark," Alex said, his voice steady with resolve, "we've built something solid here." He gestured around the well-stocked shelves and pristine counters of their pharmacy—their dream made real. "But this is just the base camp, not the peak."

Mark's attention snapped back to Alex, the entrepreneurial spark in his eyes reigniting. "I know that look," he said, a knowing grin spreading across his face. "What are you thinking?"

Alex leaned against the counter, the smooth surface cool under his palms. "We work hard for this place—make it the heart of the community. And as soon as we're able, we open another branch. We expand our reach, help more people, grow the business."

"Another branch, huh?" Mark pulled off his white pharmacist coat, hooking it onto the back of a chair. He crossed his arms, nodding slowly. "It's ambitious, but that's never stopped us before. It's what got us through exams, through late-night study sessions, and into these white coats."

"Exactly." Alex straightened up, determination etching his features. "We don't stop at survival; we aim for thrive. For us, for Sarah and Emily... for everyone who relies on us. We've come too far to slow down now."

"Then let's do it," Mark affirmed, stepping forward and extending his hand. "To the future—to our next chapter."

Their handshake was firm, an unspoken oath between them. In the quiet after-hours of their pharmacy, surrounded by the scent of antiseptics and the faint hum of refrigerators, Alex and Mark shared a moment of kinship only those who have weathered storms together could understand.

"Let's start planning," Alex said, breaking the silence. "We've got work to do."

And with the setting sun casting long shadows over their domain, they turned to the blueprints of ambition laid out before them, ready to forge ahead into the future they had promised each other ten years ago.

After a year of hard and dedicated work The bell above the pharmacy door chimed incessantly as yet another customer entered, a testament to the community's reliance and trust in the establishment Alex and Mark had built from the ground up. The shelves were meticulously stocked, and the air hummed with the quiet efficiency that had become their trademark.

"Hey, Alex," called out Mark from behind the counter, where he was consulting with an elderly man over a prescription. "We're running low on the flu shots again. People are really taking our health drives seriously."

Alex, restocking a display of vitamins, glanced over his shoulder and nodded. "I'll place another order tonight. The demand hasn't slowed down since we started offering them at cost."

"Good move, that." Mark finished counseling his patient, who left with a grateful smile. The two friends exchanged a look, one full of the silent communication honed by years of partnership.

"Another branch would mean reaching even more people," Alex mused aloud, his hands automatically straightening labels without needing to look. "We've got the support of the community here. Imagine what we could do if we bring this to another neighborhood."

"Exactly my thoughts." Mark wiped his hands on a cloth, his eyes scanning the bustling interior of their pharmacy. "We've been scouting potential locations, remember? There's that spot across town, near the new community center. It's perfect."

"More families, more kids needing vaccinations, more opportunities to educate on health and wellness." Alex's voice held the fervor of someone who believed, heart and soul, in their mission.

"Let's sit down after closing, go over the numbers one more time." Mark leaned on the counter, his entrepreneurial mind already turning over the possibilities. "If we're going to do this, we do it right. Just like we've always done."

"Agreed." Alex said, his gaze sweeping the store filled with customers—a tangible representation of their success. "We'll make it happen. More than just a business expansion, this is about impact, about being pillars in the community."

"Right there with you, partner." Mark grinned, the same excited gleam in his eyes that had sparked their journey years ago.

As the day waned and the last customer left with a wave and words of thanks, the two friends gathered their notes, spreadsheets, and the well-worn dreams they'd shared for over a decade. The shop grew quiet around them, but in their minds, the possibilities roared to life— a vision of a future not just imagined, but within their grasp, ready to be seized with the same tenacity that had carried them thus far.

The shop's neon "Closed" sign buzzed softly as Alex turned the lock, sealing them in the quiet sanctuary of their first success. He glanced back at the aisles where countless interactions had bloomed into a thriving community hub. Now, it was time for the next step. Mark pulled two chairs up to the back counter, cleared of the day's clutter, and they sank down, facing each other.

"Alright," Mark said, unfurling a city map across the counter, dotted with potential locations. "We've been over this, but once more can't hurt."

Alex leaned forward, his fingers tracing the routes between the pinned spots. "It's not just about opening another branch, Mark. It's about creating a network—a health resource that spans the city."

"Four branches," Mark echoed, his eyes bright with ambition. "That's the goal?"

"Exactly," Alex affirmed, his voice steady and sure. "Four branches in the next couple years. We'll break ground here," he tapped on a highlighted area near the burgeoning tech district, "and then spread out from there."

"Techies need flu shots too," Mark joked, yet his nod was one of approval. They understood their clientele, the ebb and flow of the city's needs, as intimately as they knew the pharmacopoeia that lined their shelves.

"Exactly," Alex repeated, a small smile creeping onto his face. "And when we say 'community pharmacy,' we mean it. Each location will be tailored to its neighborhood—its people."

"Same quality service, new addresses." Mark scribbled some figures on a notepad beside him. "It's ambitious, but then again, so were we when we started this place with barely any capital."

"Still are," Alex replied, the corner of his mouth lifting higher. The challenge fueled him, much like those late nights of study, the relentless pursuit of their licenses, the shared vision that had united them since their days dreaming in a gym locker room.

"Alright, four branches. We'll need to fine-tune our strategies, maybe bring in more staff to keep the quality consistent."

"We've got Sarah and Emily," Alex reminded him. "They've been with us every step of the way. I'm sure they'll have ideas on how we can expand without losing what makes us 'us'."

"True. And we have Maggie's support," Mark added, referring to their mentor who had given them their first shot as pharmacy assistants. "She's been invaluable."

"Remember when we were just hoping to pass that last exam?" Alex chuckled, nostalgia coloring his tone. "Now look at us, planning an empire."

"Empire is a strong word," Mark grinned. "But I like it. Let's make sure it's an empire of care, though. That's why people trust us."

"Agreed. An empire of care, then," Alex nodded solemnly before a playful glint sparked in his eye. "Starting with taking over the city one block at a time."

Leaning back, the two friends surveyed the map, their blueprint for the future. It was more than lines and names; it was a declaration of their dedication, a testament to their unyielding friendship, and a promise of prosperity and well-being for the communities they would serve. With a sense of pride and purpose, they continued poring over the details late into the night, the dream that had once felt distant now unfolding before them with each careful plan laid.

Alex stretched his arms above his head, feeling the satisfying pull of muscles that had tensed over hours of strategizing and planning. He rolled his shoulders back and let out a deep sigh, eyeing the clock on the wall—it was late, much later than he'd realized. The fluorescent lights of their makeshift conference room, a back corner of their first successful pharmacy, buzzed overhead, casting a stark contrast against the encroaching darkness outside.

"Man, we've been at this for hours," Alex remarked, his voice a mix of fatigue and excitement. He shuffled papers into a neat pile, his fingers brushing against the edges with the familiarity of someone who had lived and breathed these documents for years.

Mark nodded in agreement, his eyes still tracing the lines of the map that sprawled across the table between them—a paper battlefield where their dreams clashed with reality, each grid square a step closer to their shared goal.

"Who would've thought?" Mark mused, leaning back in his chair, the leather creaking under his weight. "From cramming for exams to plotting expansion—"

"Only the beginning, my friend," Alex interjected with a smile, his optimism unwavering even in the face of exhaustion. He stood up, pushing the chair away with the back of his legs. "But you're right. We've earned a break. Let's decompress."

"Sounds like a plan," Mark agreed, rubbing his eyes before standing up to join Alex.

"Let's grab some beer to drink from the bar," Alex suggested, his tone lightening as he envisioned the change of scenery, the clinking of glasses, and the casual banter that awaited them.

"Lead the way," Mark replied, matching Alex's lighter mood as they both exited the room.

The cool night air was refreshing after the stuffiness of their impromptu war room. They walked side by side down the empty streets, the hum of the city nightlife reaching their ears as they approached their favorite local haunt— a place where they had celebrated many small victories along the way. It was a simple bar, nothing fancy, but it held memories of their journey: the nervous laughter over pints after their first exam, the cheers when they passed, and the solemn toasts to challenges ahead.

"Here's to us," Alex said, raising his glass once they settled into their booth, the golden liquid reflecting the dim lighting of the bar.

"To us," Mark echoed, clinking his glass against Alex's, the sound sharp and clear, a harbinger of good things to come.

They drank deeply, the bitterness of the hops a perfect counterpoint to the sweetness of success, and for a moment, they allowed themselves the luxury of just being two friends, not entrepreneurs, not pharmacists—just Alex and Mark, with dreams as big as the sky above and the ambition to reach it.

Mark glanced at the antique clock above the bar, its hands creeping towards midnight. Their laughter still lingered in the air, mingling with the scent of aged wood and spilt ale. As much as he relished these moments of camaraderie, a sense of duty began to tug at him.

"Alex," Mark said, his voice cutting through the haze of their revelry, "we should get going. Our wives are waiting for us at home."

Alex nodded, the understanding between them needing no words. They stood up, leaving behind a tip that glinted like small tokens of appreciation under the bar's muted lights. The night had been a necessary release, but reality never paused for long, not even for weary dreamers.

As they donned their coats, the leather creaking softly with movement, Mark felt a twinge of anticipation for the embrace that awaited him—the warmth of home where ambition was gently shelved for love and comfort. He could already picture Sarah's soft smile, the way her eyes would light up when she saw him, reflecting all the reasons why every struggle was worth enduring.

Stepping out into the brisk night, Mark let the cool air fill his lungs, invigorating his senses. He looked over at Alex, who seemed caught in a similar reflection. Together, they started the trek back to their shared existence, the one where dreams were slowly being sculpted into reality, step by hard-earned step.

The familiar route unfolded before them, leading away from the clinking glasses and murmured conversations of the bar. Streetlights cast elongated shadows on the pavement, escorting them through the quiet city that had become the canvas for their aspirations.

"Tomorrow's another day, huh?" Alex broke the silence, a statement more than a question.

"Another day closer to everything we've worked for," Mark confirmed, feeling the weight of their upcoming ventures balanced by the support waiting at home.

Their footsteps were steady and sure—echoes of two men bound by shared goals and the unspoken pledge to weather any storm. And as the night wrapped around them, they carried within the silent promise to those they loved: they would not falter, not when so much awaited them.

After a month, The ribbon fluttered to the ground, severed by a pair of gleaming scissors in Alex's steady hand. Applause erupted from the small crowd gathered outside the new storefront, its windows gleaming with promise beneath the "Grand Opening" sign. As the clapping subsided, Alex exchanged a look with Mark, both men's faces alight with a mixture of pride and relief.

"Here we are," Mark said, his voice barely above the din of the city street, yet carrying the weight of their shared journey.

"Here we are," Alex echoed, letting his gaze sweep over the freshly painted facade of their second pharmacy branch—a tangible testament to the late nights, the sacrifices, and the unwavering resolve that had brought them to this moment.

Inside, the scent of newness—a mix of clean shelves and unspoiled carpet—greeted them like an old friend. The employees, a blend of familiar faces from their first pharmacy and eager new hires, assembled behind the checkout counters and consultation desks. They were a team, carefully chosen and ready to serve, each one a vital piece in the intricate puzzle of their burgeoning business empire.

"Welcome aboard," Alex greeted a young technician who offered him a nervous smile. "We're glad to have you with us."

"Thank you, sir," she replied, her gratitude evident. "I've heard so much about what you guys are doing here. It's exciting to be part of it."

Alex nodded, acknowledging the truth in her words. It was more than just filling prescriptions and advising on medication—it was about building a community, fostering trust, and making a difference in people's lives.

As he moved through the store, inspecting the perfectly aligned products and state-of-the-art equipment, Alex felt the hum of potential energy. This was more than a space for commerce; it was a vessel for their vision, a place where health and wellness would be championed.

Mark was already deep in conversation with the new manager, discussing logistics and operations with a focus that had become second nature to them both. Their partnership, once just two friends dreaming big, had evolved into a well-oiled machine, each knowing when to lead and when to support.

"Alright, team," Mark called out, gathering the staff with an easy authority. "Let's show our customers what we're all about. Compassion, expertise, and care—that's our promise to them. Let's deliver it every single day."

Heads nodded, a collective agreement sealed with shared determination. There was an energy in the room that couldn't be faked—an enthusiasm born of opportunity and the dawn of new beginnings.

As they stepped back onto the bustling sidewalk, Alex couldn't help but feel the thrum of life coursing through the streets—each person a story, every story a chance to make a positive impact. He looked down the road, envisioning the future branches that would one day dot the landscape like beacons.

"Two down, more to come," Alex mused aloud, a statement of intent that hung between him and Mark like a challenge eagerly accepted.

"More to come," Mark agreed, his eyes already scanning the horizon, plotting the course for their next endeavor. Together, they derived back towards their first pharmacy, ready to tackle the rest of the day's work, fueled by the adrenaline of their latest triumph—and the ceaseless drive that kept them always reaching for the next peak.

The bell above the door chimed its familiar tone as Alex flipped the sign to 'Closed'. He pulled down the window shades with a sense of finality, shutting out the last orange hues of the setting sun. Sweeping his gaze across the newly opened pharmacy, pride swelled within him at the sight of the meticulous shelves and the freshly printed labels that spelled out remedies and hope.

"Hey," Mark called from behind the counter, locking the cash register and tucking away the day's earnings. "All secure on this end."

"Great work today," Alex responded, joining Mark at the counter. His eyes roamed over the space once more, taking in every detail—the neat rows of medications, the crisp white coats of their new employees, the modern fixtures that gave the place an air of innovation. It was a tangible testament to their years of hard work and ambition.

"Thanks." Mark's voice cut through Alex's reverie. "You too, man. I mean, look at this place!"

They stood shoulder to shoulder in companionable silence, allowing themselves a brief moment to bask in the reality of their achievement. Then, with the ease of their long-standing friendship, they moved in unison toward the back office.

"Let's see how this branch will be," Alex began, pushing open the door to the small space that had become their command center.

Inside, the walls were adorned with charts and graphs depicting their business strategies and growth. "Then we can think about expanding—maybe open the third branch in another city."

Mark leaned against the desk, rubbing his chin thoughtfully. "Another city... That would definitely spread our reach. We've got a good system now; it's scalable."

"Exactly," Alex affirmed, pulling a map from the shelf and rolling it across the desk. Their fingertips brushed as they traced routes and pinpointed potential locations—a dance of dreams and decisions.

"Somewhere with a growing community, somewhere we can make a real difference," Mark suggested, tapping a finger on a promising spot.

"Agreed. We need to find the perfect balance—" Alex paused, the corner of his mouth lifting into a determined smile, "—a place that needs us just as much as we need it for our vision."

"Sounds like a plan," Mark replied, matching Alex's smile with his own. The excitement of new ventures sparked between them like a live wire.

"Let's give it a few months, gather some data, and then..." Alex's words trailed off as he looked up from the map, meeting Mark's gaze. "Then we go for it."

"Then we go for it," echoed Mark, his voice resolute, brimming with the confidence of a shared future unfolding one calculated step at a time.

The bell above the pharmacy door chimed incessantly as customers filed in and out, a testament to the burgeoning success of Alex and Mark's second branch. The shelves were stocked with precision, labels out, every product gleaming under the bright fluorescent lights. Pharmacists, clad in crisp white coats, navigated the aisles with ease, offering smiles and knowledgeable advice.

"Can you believe this, Mark?" Alex murmured, leaning on the counter, his eyes tracking the steady flow of patrons. "Six months... It feels like just yesterday we were sketching out ideas on napkins at that diner."

Mark, busy reviewing a prescription, glanced up, his expression one of both pride and mild disbelief. "I know," he replied, cap affixed back on the pen with a satisfying click. "Word-of-mouth has done wonders for us. It's not just

about the meds; it's how we make them feel—
the community trusts us."

"Exactly." Alex straightened up, nodding to an
elderly couple as they approached. "Good
afternoon, Mr. and Mrs. Jennings. Refill on the
usual?"

"Indeed," chuckled Mr. Jennings, his arm
looped through his wife's. "We'd go nowhere
else, Alex. You boys always take such good
care of us."

"Thank you, that means the world to us," Alex
said warmly, punching in details into the
computer. He handed over the neatly bagged
items, his fingers brushing against their
weathered hands—a silent promise of care.

As the couple shuffled away, content with their
service, Mark joined Alex behind the counter,
watching the scene unfold. "They're right,
though. We've worked hard to create a place
that's more than transactions—it's about
connections."

"Which reminds me," Alex began, retrieving a
stack of loyalty cards. "Let's start handing
these out. A little thank you for their support.
Might be old-fashioned, but people appreciate
the gesture."

"Old-fashioned works," Mark agreed, taking half the stack. "It's personal, and that's what sets us apart."

Throughout the day, they met with regulars, greeted newcomers, and handled every question with unwavering patience. Their demeanor never wavered from genuine kindness—a stark contrast to the cold efficiency often found elsewhere.

As the sun dipped below the horizon, casting long shadows across the newly swept floors, Alex locked the doors with a satisfied sigh. Side by side, they stood, peering through the glass at the quiet street outside.

"Look at us, huh?" Mark said, a hint of awe threading his voice. "Two guys with a dream, and now look—people know us, trust us. That's real wealth, Alex."

"More branches to come," Alex added, slinging an arm around Mark's shoulders. "But let's savor this moment. This isn't just business; it's our life's work."

"Here's to treating people right," Mark raised an imaginary toast, "and to the future."

"Cheers to that," Alex echoed, grinning broadly. With a shared nod, they turned off the lights, their aspirations as luminous as the stars beginning to twinkle in the twilight sky.

The evening air was crisp, hinting at the arrival of night as Alex turned the key in the ignition of his modest sedan. The car's engine hummed softly, a background melody to the thoughts swirling in his head. He glanced over to Mark, who was already pulling out of the pharmacy parking lot beside him. Both vehicles eased onto the road, parting ways with a casual honk, their paths lit by the glow of streetlamps.

Alex's mind lingered on the day's successes, the warmth of each interaction at the pharmacy filling him with a quiet pride. As he drove through familiar streets, the storefronts and houses faded into blurs of color. His focus was on the home that awaited him, the soft light from the windows promising solace after the day's toil.

Pulling into the driveway, he killed the engine and sat for a moment in the silence, savoring the stillness. He ran his fingers through his hair, which had grown slightly longer than usual, a testament to the dedication that left little time for personal grooming. With a deep breath, he gathered his belongings and stepped out into the night.

At the front door, he paused, a smile curving his lips as he heard soft laughter from within—Sarah's laughter, a sound that had become a beacon of joy in his life. He let himself in, the warmth of the house embracing him like an old friend. Sarah looked up from where she sat on the couch, her eyes brightening.

"Hey, ambitious man," she greeted, her voice laced with affectionate teasing. "How's our favorite pharmacist?"

"Exhausted, but good," Alex replied, setting his bag down and bending to kiss her forehead. "The second branch is thriving, love. It's all coming together."

"Come sit. You need to rest," Sarah patted the cushion next to her, a gentle command he couldn't refuse.

He obliged, sinking into the couch with a contented sigh. Sarah nestled against him, her presence a balm to the day's remnants of stress. They spoke little, the tranquility between them saying more than words ever could. In the shared silence, Alex found the peace he didn't know he needed.

As the clock chimed late into the night, they rose together, a synchronous dance born of intimate familiarity. Sarah led him to their bedroom, where the promise of rest beckoned. There, entwined in the soft sheets and each other's arms, sleep came easily, a well-deserved reprieve for two souls united in love and ambition.

The morning light filtered through the curtains, casting a golden glow over the breakfast nook where Alex sat, sipping his coffee. He leafed through a stack of supplier invoices, his mind half on the numbers and half on the rhythmic chirping of the birds outside.

A knock on the door broke his concentration. He glanced at the clock; it was early for visitors. Setting his mug down, he walked to the front door and opened it to find Mark standing there, a grin splitting his face and a rolled-up architectural magazine in his hand.

"Morning, partner," Mark said, stepping into the house without waiting for an invitation. "Hope I didn't wake you."

"Already up," Alex replied, closing the door. "What's got you bouncing this early?"

Mark tapped the magazine against his palm, excitement sparking in his eyes. "I've been thinking, Alex. We're on track for the third branch, and with the way things are going, the fourth won't be far behind."

Alex nodded, intrigued by Mark's enthusiasm. "Go on."

"Once we open that fourth pharmacy," Mark continued, unfurling the magazine to reveal glossy pages of grand estates and luxurious mansions, "let's buy a house like a castle and live there together. Think about it—a testament to our success, a place big enough for both our families, where we can host gatherings and enjoy the fruits of our labor."

For a moment, Alex was silent, absorbing the idea. The notion seemed lavish, almost fantastical, but then again, hadn't their entire journey been a chase after a dream? A shared vision that had started in the depths of failure and bloomed into something tangible?

"Live like kings in a castle, huh?" Alex said with a chuckle, his entrepreneurial spirit ignited by the challenge. "That's quite the ambition. But after everything we've achieved, why not?"

"Exactly!" Mark slapped the magazine onto the table. "We set out to make something of ourselves, not just to get by. It's more than just a place to live. It's a statement, a haven for our future."

Alex picked up the magazine, thumbing through the pages, allowing himself to envision walking through grand halls and manicured gardens. It was bold, it was audacious—it was precisely the kind of goal they had always set for themselves.

"Let's do it," Alex said firmly, meeting Mark's gaze with a determined glint in his own. "Let's work towards our castle."

Mark's smile widened, mirroring Alex's resolve. They had come so far from those days of doubt and uncertainty. This new dream would be another chapter in their story, a narrative of two friends who dared to aim higher, time and time again.

The morning light filtered through the kitchen blinds, casting a warm glow over the breakfast table where Alex and Mark sat with their wives. Mugs of coffee steamed in their hands as they engaged in the comfortable chatter that comes with shared history and friendship.

"Sarah, Em," Alex began, his tone carrying an excited undertone, "Mark and I have been talking about something." He exchanged a glance with Mark, who nodded encouragingly.

"Go on," Sarah prompted, her curiosity piqued as she tucked a loose strand of hair behind her ear.

"We've been thinking, once we open our fourth pharmacy," Mark said, pausing for dramatic effect, "we want to buy a house. But not just any house—a place that's grand, like a castle, where we can all live together."

The words hung in the air, a daring proposition that seemed to hover between fantasy and reality. Alex watched as the expressions on Sarah and Emily's faces morphed from surprise to contemplation.

"A castle?" Emily repeated, her voice tinged with amusement. "You boys really do dream big."

"Think about it," Alex said, leaning forward. "It would be more than a home. It'd be a symbol of everything we've worked for, a testament to our dedication. And we'd share it with the two most important people in our lives."

The women exchanged looks, their eyes communicating in that silent language only close companions understand. Sarah's lips curved into a smile that lit up her face. "I love it," she said, the enthusiasm in her voice genuine. "I mean, why not? We've seen what you both are capable of, and if anyone can turn such a bold dream into reality, it's you two."

"Absolutely," Emily chimed in, reaching across the table to give Mark's hand an affectionate squeeze. "You've already built so much from the ground up. A castle for our families... it sounds like a fairy tale, but one I'd be happy to step into."

Mark's eyes sparkled with joy and relief. Alex felt a surge of warmth at the approval; their shared vision now included the women they loved, making it all the more precious.

"Then it's settled," Alex declared, his voice buoyant with optimism. "We'll work towards our castle, not just for us, but for our family."

"Here's to the next chapter," Mark raised his mug in a toast.

"To castles and dreams," Sarah added, her voice filled with excitement.

"To family," Emily concluded, the four of them clinking their mugs together in a chorus of ceramic meeting ceramic, sealing their collective ambition with the simple act.

couple months later, The morning air was crisp, carrying the scent of fresh ambition as Alex turned the key in the lock of their third pharmacy. The metallic click echoed through the stillness of the empty shop, a prelude to the bustling days ahead. With a gentle nudge, the door swung open, and sunlight poured onto the pristine white tiles, casting long shadows behind the shelves that stood eager to be stocked.

"Here we are," Mark said, stepping inside and running a hand along the counter's smooth surface. His eyes held a glimmer of pride, reflecting years of hard-earned success.

Alex nodded, his gaze sweeping over the interior. Each corner of the space was a testament to their relentless drive, the late nights pouring over financial plans, and the early mornings restocking and preparing for the day's customers. This was more than a business; it was a physical manifestation of their tenacity, a symbol of the dreams they were steadily turning into reality.

"Can't believe this is number three," Alex murmured, taking in the expanse of the store. It was larger than the previous two, with wider aisles and a prominent consultation area that spoke of their commitment to customer care.

"Believe it," Mark replied, patting Alex on the back. "We've come a long way from cramming for exams and dreaming about what could be."

"Remember how we used to talk about making an impact?" Alex's voice was thick with nostalgia as he gestured toward the space designated for community health education. "Looks like we're really doing it, huh?"

"More than that," Mark agreed. "We're building something lasting, not just for us, but for everyone who walks through those doors."

They moved together through the pharmacy, each turn an affirmation of their partnership. They discussed the placement of products, the flow of customer traffic, and the integration of technology to streamline operations—an interplay of ideas that had become as natural as breathing.

"Next up, the grand opening," Alex said, the excitement surging in his chest.

"Yep, and then onto planning branch number four," Mark added, a grin spreading across his face. "Still aiming for that castle?"

"Always," Alex affirmed, his smile mirroring Mark's. They had learned to balance their graft with grandeur, never losing sight of the horizon even while their hands worked the soil.

"Let's get to it, then," Mark said, rolling up his sleeves. "There's no rest for the ambitious."

"Or for dreamers," Alex added, lifting a box filled with supplies from the floor, muscles tensing with the weight.

"Especially not for dreamers who do," Mark concluded, taking up a box of his own.

Together, they began stocking the shelves, each item placed a step further on their journey. Outside, the city carried on, unaware of the small miracle unfolding within the walls of the new pharmacy. But for Alex and Mark, the world was exactly where they stood—between aisles and aspirations, on the cusp of their next great venture.

The first rays of morning light filtered through the freshly cleaned windows, casting a warm glow over the polished countertops of the new pharmacy. Alex surveyed the space with pride, the scent of disinfectant and new paint lingering in the air as Mark unpacked a box of brochures detailing their community health initiatives.

"Same layout as the first two?" Alex asked, his hands gesturing to the shelves that would soon be lined with medicines and wellness products.

"Absolutely," Mark replied without missing a beat, smoothing out a crease in one of the pamphlets. "Consistency is key. Our customers should feel at home in any of our locations."

Alex nodded, his thoughts aligning perfectly with Mark's. They had built a reputation not just on the quality of their products but on the integrity of their service. Every smile, every piece of advice, every effort to go above and beyond for those who walked through their doors—it was these threads that wove the fabric of their growing enterprise.

"Let's make sure our staff training emphasizes that," Alex said, placing a hand on the counter. "The personal touch—that's what sets us apart."

"Got it." Mark set down the brochure and picked up his tablet to make a note. "Honesty, care, compassion. It's what got us here, and it's what'll keep us going."

They moved in sync, Alex arranging the displays while Mark updated their training protocols, each action reinforcing the shared vision that had propelled them from dreamers to achievers. It wasn't just about filling prescriptions; it was about fostering relationships, about being a cornerstone of the neighborhood.

Mark looked up, a reminiscent twinkle in his eye. "And now we're here, setting up shop number three." He shook his head in disbelief. "Feels good, doesn't it?"

"Better than good," Alex affirmed, stepping back to survey their handiwork. "It feels right."

In the heart of the pharmacy, surrounded by the tangible results of their relentless dedication, the two friends shared a moment of quiet satisfaction. Beyond the glass door, the world continued its relentless spin, but inside, they had created an oasis of trust and care—a testament to their unwavering commitment to their craft and their community.

The bell above the pharmacy door tinkled, a familiar sound that Alex had grown to associate with progress and community. He glanced up from the prescription he was filling for Mrs. Henderson, his eyes meeting those of an elderly man who shuffled in, leaning heavily on a carved wooden cane.

"Good afternoon, Mr. Bartlett," Alex greeted, his voice warm with recognition.

"Alex, my boy," the old man replied, his face folding into a smile that belied the years etched into his skin. "I've come to make a decision, one I hope sits well with you."

Alex nodded, excusing himself from the counter to approach Mr. Bartlett more closely. Mark, from across the room, caught sight of the interaction and drifted over, sensing the gravity of the moment.

"Go on, sir," Alex encouraged, as Mark arrived at his side.

Mr. Bartlett's grip tightened around the handle of his cane. "I've watched you boys," he began, his voice carrying the weight of many winters, "turn this place into more than just a business. It's a sanctuary—a place where healing begins before medicine is even dispensed."

Mark exchanged a glance with Alex, both feeling a swell of pride. It was precisely what they had strived for.

"Thank you, Mr. Bartlett," Mark said. "That means everything to us."

"Which brings me to my point." The old man took a deep breath, steadying himself. "I'm retiring, lads. My own little shop has seen better days, and I reckon it's time to pass the baton. I want you two to have it."

Alex felt a jolt of surprise, quickly followed by a surge of opportunity. Their third pharmacy had thrived under the same principles that had guided their first two, and now the chance to expand further lay before them.

"Are you sure?" Alex asked gently. Mr. Bartlett had been a pillar of the pharmaceutical community for decades; his store was a local institution.

"Never been surer," Mr. Bartlett confirmed. "I've had offers, but I want it in hands that value more than the bottom line. I want a legacy of care."

Mark stepped forward, extending his hand. "We'd be honored, Mr. Bartlett. We'll carry on your legacy with every ounce of integrity you've shown."

"Then it's settled." A look of relief washed over the old man's features. "Come by tomorrow, we'll sort the details. But for now..." He took a step back, observing the bustling pharmacy around him. "I think I'll sit and enjoy the view one last time as owner."

"Of course, take all the time you need," Alex said, motioning towards a comfortable chair near the consultation area.

As Mr. Bartlett settled into the chair, his gaze lingering on the interactions between staff and customers, Alex and Mark stood shoulder to shoulder, their vision expanding with each beat of their entrepreneurial hearts.

"Four pharmacies, Mark," Alex whispered, almost in awe. "Can you believe it?"

"Believe it? I can see it," Mark replied, a determined glint in his eye. "This is just the beginning, Alex. Just the beginning."

Together, they turned back to their work, the future unfurling before them like a well-read map, every line and contour leading to new horizons, new communities to serve, and dreams realized.

after a while, Alex leaned his back against the cool glass of the front window of their latest acquisition, the fourth pharmacy, and watched Mark flip through the final pages of the contract. The fluorescent lights hummed overhead, casting a clinical glow over the counters lined with medications, bandages, and health brochures.

"Here," Mark said, tapping a clause in the document. "This is it—the culmination of our hard work."

"Indeed," Alex agreed, pushing off from the window to join his friend. He took the pen that Mark offered and, with a steady hand, signed his name beside Mark's on the dotted line. The ink felt permanent, symbolic—a testament to their years of relentless pursuit.

"Four pharmacies," Alex mused, setting down the pen. He looked around at the shelves stocked full of remedies and aids, thinking of all the people they would help, all the lives that would intersect with theirs in this space. "Remember when we were just dreaming about this moment? Studying late into the night, believing that one day it would all be worth it?"

"Every sacrifice, every obstacle," Mark added, a note of pride threading his voice. "We've built something tangible, something good."

"Exactly." Alex clapped a hand on Mark's shoulder, sharing a smile steeped in camaraderie and shared ambition. "And now, my friend, I think it's time for us to claim our reward. Not just these walls and counters, but the life we dreamed up when this journey began."

Mark's eyes lit up with understanding, and he nodded. "The castle," he said, the word itself carrying the weight of their aspirations.

"Let's stop here," Alex stated firmly, his gaze locking with Mark's. "Let's buy this pharmacy, so we have four pharmacies now, and let's buy the castle and enjoy our life."

The idea hung between them, rich with possibility. They had climbed tirelessly, reached the peak of one mountain, and now it was time to bask in the view before seeking new summits.

"Enjoy our life," Mark repeated, as if tasting the words, savoring the flavor of leisure after the long feast of labor.

"Let's do it," Alex affirmed with a decisive nod. "Let's live the life we've worked for, side by side with the people we love. Let's create a home that's as grand as our dreams."

"Agreed," Mark said, his voice resolute. "We've earned it, and more importantly, we'll share it—with Sarah, with Emily, with everyone who's been part of this adventure."

Their laughter echoed in the empty store, a sound full of promise and future joys. The dream of a castle was no longer a mere silhouette on the horizon; it was real, reachable, and ready to be filled with memories yet to be made.

"Let's start the next chapter," Alex suggested, the excitement bubbling within him.

"Right behind you," replied Mark, already reaching for his phone to make the arrangements.

As they stepped out of the pharmacy, the first step toward their castle taken, the sun dipped low in the sky, painting their path in hues of gold and amber—a fitting end to a day that marked a new beginning.

Sitting in the back room of their newest acquisition, Alex and Mark faced each other across a cluttered desk. The walls around them bore the marks of a long history, whispering secrets of health restored and comfort provided. Now, they were ready to write the next chapter—their own.

"Okay, it's decided then," Alex said, tapping his fingers on the desktop. "We find someone to manage all four pharmacies. Someone we trust to run things just like we would."

Mark ran a hand through his hair, nodding. His eyes gleamed with the reflection of the computer screen as he scrolled through resumes. "Absolutely. We've been hands-on from day one, but it's time to delegate. We need someone with the same drive, the same commitment to community service."

"Exactly." Alex leaned back, stretching his arms. "Someone who understands that these aren't just stores; they're lifelines to the people."

Their search was meticulous, each candidate's profile reviewed with the precision they had applied to their studies, their work, their very lives. They combed through qualifications, experience, testimonials, searching for the person who could carry their legacy forward.

At last, they found a resume that stood out—a blend of experience and passion that mirrored their own journey. Mark pointed at the screen, excitement building in his chest. "This one. This person has worked in community pharmacies for over a decade, has an entrepreneurial spirit, and volunteers on weekends. They get it."

"Let's set up an interview," Alex replied, his decision-making as sharp as ever. He could already envision walking away from the daily grind, trusting that their hard-earned empire was in capable hands.

"Imagine, Alex," Mark said, his voice hushed with the gravity of their new reality. "We can actually start living more. No more late nights restocking shelves or covering shifts. Just... life."

"Searching for our castle," Alex mused, allowing himself a rare moment to daydream. "Can you picture it? A grand estate, maybe with a view of the lake, where we can host barbecues for our friends, have space for kids to play..."

"Family gatherings, holidays..." Mark added, caught up in the vision. "The kind of home that becomes a sanctuary, not just for us but for everyone we love."

"Exactly," Alex said, a smile spreading across his face. "A home that's more than just stone and wood—it's a symbol. Of everything we've achieved, everything we've overcome."

"Then let's do it," Mark said, determination firm in his voice. "Let's take this step back so we can enjoy the life we've built."

"Agreed," Alex replied, feeling the weight of responsibility begin to lift. "We'll hire the manager and start the hunt for our castle. It's time."

And with that, they shook hands—partners in business, brothers in spirit—ready to embark on the most rewarding adventure yet: the quest for a place to call not just a house, but a forever home.

Alex leaned back in the leather chair, a sense of contentment washing over him as he perused the glossy brochures strewn across the mahogany desk. Each page revealed sprawling estates nestled in verdant landscapes, turrets piercing the sky, and long, winding driveways that promised a journey to somewhere magical.

"Look at this one," Mark said, pointing to an image of a majestic castle surrounded by acres of woodland. The reflection of the setting sun turned its windows into panels of gold. "It has a private lake."

"Perfect for those summer getaways we always talked about," Alex replied, envisioning their future gatherings, laughter echoing against the high ceilings, the clinking of glasses on the terrace as dusk settled in.

They had come a long way from their humble beginnings, from late-night study sessions and dreams scribbled on coffee-stained napkins. Now, with the decision to hire a manager for their pharmacies, a new chapter was unfolding—one with fewer prescriptions and more possibilities.

"We could have our own forest, a place to disconnect," Alex mused, his finger tracing the outline of a wooded trail on the brochure. "A sanctuary away from the buzz of the city."

"True," Mark agreed, his eyes gleaming with anticipation. "We can finally enjoy the fruits of our labor. Imagine waking up to the sound of birds instead of alarm clocks."

"Exactly." Alex closed his eyes for a moment, allowing himself to be transported by the thought. "And when we find the right place, it will be more than just walls—it'll be the heart of our legacy."

Mark nodded, a silent pact forming between them. This wasn't just about luxury or status; it was about creating a home where their past struggles would be honored and their future joy secured.

"Let's schedule some visits," Mark suggested, picking up the phone to call the real estate agent. "It's time we took a proper look at what our next big dream is made of."

"Couldn't agree more," Alex said, standing up. Together, they stepped out onto the balcony overlooking the city they had conquered, ready to conquer yet another realm—the realm of their grandest dreams.

couple days later,The wind tousled Alex's hair as he leaned out of the passenger window, drinking in the crisp air that swept across the serene lakeshore. Emerald waves lapped at the pebbles, a rhythmic melody that promised peace. Beside him, Sarah's eyes sparkled with shared excitement, her hand squeezing his every time a new silhouette of a castle appeared on the horizon.

"Look at that one," she whispered, pointing to a grand structure nestled between two hills, its reflection shimmering in the water like a mirage of their aspirations.

"Let's hope the inside is as promising as the view," Alex replied, a grin spreading across his face.

In the backseat, Mark and Emily were huddled close, poring over glossy printouts of property listings, their murmurs a hum of hopeful speculation. Every so often, Emily would laugh—a clear, bell-like sound that reminded Alex of their college days, when dreams were plentiful and worries scarce.

The real estate agent, a woman with an air of efficiency, navigated the winding road with practiced ease. "We'll be approaching the first location shortly," she announced, glancing at them in the rearview mirror. "It's quite secluded, perfect for those who value privacy."

As they turned onto a gravel path flanked by towering pines, a sense of anticipation coursed through Alex. The trees parted like curtains revealing a stage, and there it was—their potential future home, a castle perched at the lake's edge, its stone façade kissed by sunlight.

"Wow," Mark breathed out, leaning forward. "It's like something out of a fairytale."

"Let's explore," Alex said, the words barely out before they were all unfastening seat belts and spilling out of the car.

They approached the castle, footsteps crunching on the gravel, each step amplifying their eagerness. The real estate agent retrieved the key from a lockbox, the metallic click echoing their racing pulses.

"Ready?" she asked, pushing open the heavy oak door.

The interior unveiled itself, a dance of shadow and light played out in the vast hall. Stained glass windows painted the floor in vibrant hues, and for a moment, they all stood silent, lost in the beauty of it all.

"Imagine the kids running around here," Sarah murmured, her gaze softening as she envisioned a future filled with laughter and warmth.

"Or the parties we could throw," Emily added, her voice tinged with the thrill of social gatherings yet to come.

"First things first," Alex interjected, the businessman within surfacing. "We need to make sure it's structurally sound, energy-efficient. This isn't just a home; it's an investment."

"Always the pragmatist," Mark teased, but his eyes held respect. They both knew the importance of practicality, especially after years of hard work and careful planning.

"Let's see the rest," Alex suggested, leading the way deeper into the castle.

As they explored room after room, each space whispered secrets of a bygone era, beckoning them to write their own history within these ancient walls. The laughter of the group bounced off vaulted ceilings, filling the empty spaces with life once more.

Standing at the edge of a balcony, Alex wrapped an arm around Sarah, and together they gazed out at the lake, its surface a tapestry of undulating colors beneath the setting sun.

"Could this be it?" Sarah asked, her voice barely above a whisper.

"Maybe," Alex replied. "But let's not decide too quickly. We have more castles to see."

"Of course," she agreed, but her smile told him she was already half in love with this place.

They lingered a moment longer, letting the tranquility seep into their bones before regrouping with the others to discuss thoughts and impressions.

"Next stop?" Mark asked, ready to continue their quest.

"Next stop," Alex confirmed, a leader among equals.

Together, they left the castle behind, the image of its grandeur etched into their collective memory, a contender in the race to become the cornerstone of their new lives.

The real estate agent's glossy brochure had promised a day of wonder, a feast for the eyes with an array of lakeside castles, each more breathtaking than the last. Yet as the sun dipped lower in the sky, casting long shadows over their path, Alex couldn't shake the image of the first one from his mind.

"Look at this one, with the turrets reaching up like it's trying to touch the clouds," Emily pointed out as they toured another grand estate, her voice tinged with awe.

"Beautiful, yes," Mark conceded, stepping back to take in the view. "But it doesn't have the same... I don't know, the same heart?"

"Agreed," Alex said. "It feels too cold, too impersonal."

Their procession continued through manicured gardens and echoing halls, but the magic was absent. The laughter that had filled the first castle's rooms had dulled to polite murmurs. They were going through the motions, ticking off boxes on a list that no longer held meaning.

"Guys," Sarah began, her hand slipping into Alex's, "remember the balcony overlooking the lake at the first place? How peaceful it felt?"

"Exactly," Alex replied. "None of these have matched that feeling."

"Should we...?" Mark left the question hanging, but his gaze met Alex's with understanding.

"Let's go back to the first one," Alex decided, the resolve clear in his voice. It wasn't just about walls and location; it was about envisioning their future, picturing their families growing amidst those old stones, breathing new life into them.

"Really?" Emily's face lit up, her previous reservations fading. "I loved the kitchen there. It had such a warm, lived-in feel."

"Back to the beginning then," the real estate agent chirped, masking her surprise with practiced ease. "Sometimes the heart knows before the mind catches up."

The decision made, they retraced their steps, leaving behind the parade of properties that lacked the intangible essence they all yearned for. As they returned to the first castle, the sense of rightness settled over Alex like a comforting blanket.

They walked through the arched doorway once again, and it was as if the castle itself greeted them back, the rays of the setting sun like golden ribbons welcoming them home.

Stepping over the threshold, Alex's eyes adjusted to the grandeur of the entry hall, its walls echoing with the gentle hush of their footsteps. Mark followed close behind, his hand resting lightly on Emily's back. They wandered into the expansive living room, where the last rays of the setting sun painted the space in a soft amber glow.

"Can you believe we're standing here?" Alex murmured, his voice tinged with awe as he ran his fingers along the mantle of the fireplace.

Mark chuckled, a sound of triumph mixed with nostalgia. "From cramming for exams in that tiny apartment to this," he gestured around the vast room, "it's surreal."

Sarah nestled closer to Alex, her presence a reminder of the unwavering support they had received. "You two have come so far," she said softly. "There were moments I wasn't sure we'd make it through. All those nights studying and working doubles..."

Emily nodded in agreement, her eyes meeting Mark's with a mixture of pride and affection. "But look at what you've built because of it. Your dedication... It's inspiring."

Alex caught Sarah's gaze, gratitude welling up within him. "We couldn't have done it without you girls." He reached out, capturing her hand in his. "You were our rock when everything felt like it was crumbling."

"More than once," Mark added, "I thought about giving up. But then I'd see Emily's notes in the margins of my textbooks, little reminders that kept me pushing forward."

They moved together, gravitating towards the large bay window that offered a view of the tranquil lake. The water reflected the changing colors of the sky, a testament to the passage of time and the fluidity of life's journey.

"Every step, every setback, it was all worth it," Alex said, his voice filled with conviction. "To stand here now, with all of you, ready to start this new chapter."

"Remember when we lived off instant ramen and dreamed of days like this?" Mark laughed, the sound mingling with the quiet lapping of the lake's waters against the shore.

"Those dreams fueled us," Sarah replied, squeezing Alex's hand. "And now they're our reality."

"Here's to never surrendering," Emily said, lifting an imaginary glass.

"To dreams coming true," Alex echoed, his heart full as he looked around at the faces of those he loved most.

The castle, grand and imposing, stood silent around them, its walls bearing witness to the culmination of their journey—a journey not just of ambition and success, but of love, friendship, and the unyielding belief in one another.

Standing shoulder to shoulder, Alex and Mark surveyed the castle's grand hall, the air rich with the scent of aged wood and the promise of new beginnings. They had traversed the rugged road to success together, each challenge a stepping stone towards this very moment.

"Hey," Alex said, his voice soft yet steady, "I could never have done this without you, man." He turned to face Mark, gratitude shining in his eyes. "You've been more than a friend; you're my brother."

Mark met Alex's gaze, an understanding smile tugging at his lips. "We've both come so far," he responded, his arm reaching out to clasp Alex's shoulder. "Brothers indeed – by choice, not by blood. We chose this path together."

A comfortable silence settled between them, laden with shared memories of late nights studying, endless shifts, and the unwavering support that carried them through. It was more than friendship; it was a bond forged in the fires of shared ambition and mutual respect.

Finally, they turned their attention back to the room, where Sarah and Emily waited expectantly, their support having been pivotal in the duo's journey. The women's eyes held a reflection of the pride mirrored in Alex and Mark's hearts.

"Let's do it then," Alex announced, his voice resonating with certainty. "This is more than just a house. It's a symbol of everything we've achieved and everything we'll continue to build."

"Agreed," Mark chimed in, nodding decisively. "We've worked too hard to settle for anything less than our dream."

The decision hung in the air, weighty and significant. They all knew that purchasing this castle meant more than acquiring property; it represented the manifestation of years of sacrifice and dedication, a tangible reminder that dreams, no matter how vast, were within their grasp.

"Let's go live our happy life," Sarah whispered, her words a gentle nudge towards the future.

"Let's," Emily echoed, her voice vibrant with excitement.

With a collective inhale, the four of them stood united, ready to cross the threshold into a new era. They stepped forward, hand in hand, hearts intertwined, embarking on the next grand adventure that life had to offer, surrounded by the walls of their new home—a castle fit for the kings and queens of their own making.

Alex stepped toward the grand window, his gaze sweeping over the expanse of the glistening lake beyond. The sun dipped low, sending ripples of gold dancing across the water, echoing the promise of a new dawn. He turned to the others, eyes alight with the fiery determination that had fueled their journey.

"Can you imagine waking up to this every day?" Alex's voice broke the reflective silence, each word infused with dreams crystallized into reality.

Mark joined him at the window, a grin spreading across his face as he envisioned their future. "I've imagined it for years, and now it's right in front of us."

Sarah and Emily approached, their arms looping around their partners'. A shared look passed between them—a look of enduring love and unwavering support for the men they had championed through every high and low.

"Let's make this our sanctuary," Sarah said, her tone laced with warmth and the comfort of a long journey finally at its rest.

"An oasis where we can grow old, watch seasons change, and build a lifetime of memories," added Emily, her words painting pictures of the future gatherings, laughter, and the legacy they would create within these walls.

"Are we all in agreement then?" Mark asked, but it was more a formality than a question. The bond they shared, solidified through struggle and success, needed no further affirmation.

"Absolutely," Alex replied, the hint of a smile tugging at his lips. "This is our next chapter."

"Then it's decided," Mark declared, his voice resonating with finality. "We're buying it."

They turned to each other, the connection between them palpable. Each pair exchanged a glance, an unspoken vow of commitment not just to the house, but to the life they would build together.

"Let's go live our happy life," Alex said, his heart swelling with pride and contentment. It was a simple statement, yet it held the weight of their shared history and the boundless hope of their collective future.

"Let's," they all agreed in unison, voices mingling together in the spacious room that would soon be filled with the echoes of their continued adventures.

With a sense of unity and anticipation, they clasped hands, stepping out of the shadow of their past and into the luminous glow of their happily ever after. They walked through the castle that was to be their home, each step a testament to their resilience, their friendship, and the love that had become the cornerstone of their extraordinary lives.

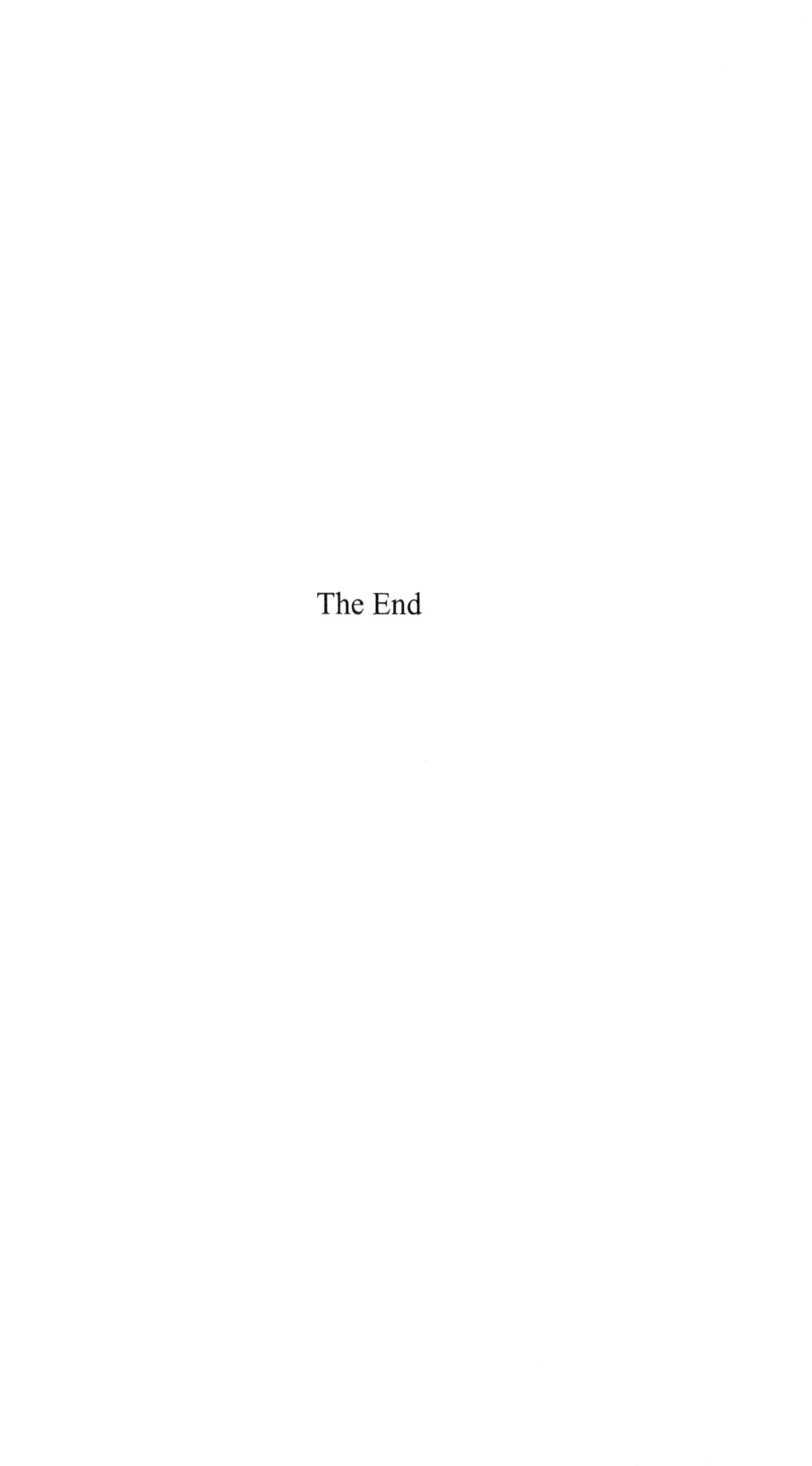

The End

Now, do you think that you can do the same?

Ask yourself:

 Do you wish to become rich, or you are obligated to do so?

Do you think you are getting closer to your goal?

When you think about your goal do you think you are on the right path?

Keep your answers on your mind and here are some tips for you:

Never give up no matter how many times you fail.

Don't talk about your dream to anyone.

Keep going straight and don't turn to the Distractions.

Control yourself, your emotions and your feelings.

Wish good for people and help them as much as you can because selfishness is the basis of failure.

Choose the right partner to spend your life with because this may determine 100% of your happiness.

Also, Self-love is the most important thing, without it you can't do anything

9 798300 314064